Excerpts from
The MEDICAL and NUTRITIONAL APPROACH To HYPERTENSION

Hypertension is not a disease . . . it is a symptom and its importance depends on the significance of its cause.　　　Chapter 1

* * *

Quickie meals at fast-food fare restaurants and the race for material possessions are contributory causes of high blood pressure.

Chapter 2

* * *

It is often said that blood pressure should normally measure *"100 plus your age,"* and that *"low blood pressure"* is a dangerous condition. Neither of these notions are true.　　　Chapter 4

* * *

Salt intake and excessive weight contribute to hypertension. High Blood Pressure affects three areas of the body.　　　Chapter 6

* * *

Tranquilizers are often prescribed for High Blood Pressure. But nature's tranquilizer has far fewer side effects.　　　Chapter 7

* * *

Dr. Rinse developed a *"breakfast mash"* that freed him from symptoms of heart and circulatory problems and increased his energy level.

Chapter 8

* * *

Some have termed Garlic not only *"the fountain of youth"* but nature's way of lowering blood pressure effectively and safely.

Chapter 13

* * *

One of the　B　vitamins, researchers claim, is the best safeguard against heart disease and blood pressure problems.　　　Chapter 15

* * *

Some nutritionists strongly believe the answer to high blood pressure is found in first having a hair analysis and then following a personalized vitamin/mineral supplement program.　　　Chapter 17

* * *

All this and <u>much more</u> you will find in the chapters of this revealing book on *The Medical Approach versus The Nutritional Approach To High Blood Pressure!*

Important Legal Notice

The Medical Approach
versus
The Nutritional Approach
To
HIGH BLOOD PRESSURE

by Salem Kirban

Published by SALEM KIRBAN, Inc., Kent Road, Huntingdon Valley, Pennsylvania 19006. Copyright © 1982 by Salem Kirban. Printed in United States of America. All rights reserved, including the right to reproduce this book or portions thereof in any form.

Library of Congress Catalog Card No. 81-84440
ISBN 0-912582-45-6

ACKNOWLEDGMENTS

To **Estelle Bair Composition** for excellent craftsmanship in setting type.

To **Walter W. Slotilock,** Chapel Hill Litho, for negatives.

To **Bob Jackson,** for illustrations on pages 21, 24, 33, 34 ,35 38, 42, 43.

To **Dickinson Brothers, Inc.,** for printing this book.

And special thanks to the following publishers for graciously making available medical illustrations for this book:

Intermed Communications, Inc., Springhouse, Pennsylvania 19477
Illustrations reprinted with permission from Diseases, Copyright © 1981.

J.B. Lippincott Company, Philadelphia, Pennsylvania 19105
Illustrations reprinted with permission from Textbook of Medical-Surgical Nursing by L. Brunner and D. Suddarth, ed. 4, Copyright © 1980.

Mitchell Beazley Publishers, Ltd., England
Atlas of the Body and Mind, Copyright ©Mitchell Beazley Publishers, Ltd. 1976. Published in U.S.A. by **Rand McNally & Company.**

Life & Health Magazine
For illustration on page 28.

CONTENTS

Special Features Include

HOW TO READ LABELS

Too much salt in your system affects the nerves of your stomach and causes food to cling to the walls of your colon. The intestine loses its elasticity and stretches. The Tranverse Colon (the horizontal portion), begins to sag giving you a noticeable protruding stomach. Calcium and potassium depleted to dangerous levels.

For your life ... it is important, therefore, that you know how to read supermarket labels found on the foods you purchase.

The labels of most foods must list what is in them ... <u>in order of predominance by weight</u> – the <u>main</u> ingredient <u>first</u>, the <u>next</u> most plentiful <u>second</u>, etc. Many food manufacturers are reluctant to list sodium or salt content of foods because of the public's increasing awareness to nutrition ... and because the adding of salt does encourage increased sales.

Be sure to read the labels and look for the words <u>SODIUM</u> or any word that has sodium as part of its name. Also beware of <u>MSG</u> (monosodium glutamate). It is a form of salt!

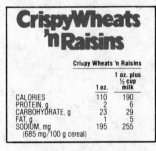

Crispy Wheats 'n Raisins

	1 oz.	1 oz. plus ½ cup milk
CALORIES	110	190
PROTEIN, g	2	6
CARBOHYDRATE, g	23	29
FAT, g	1	5
SODIUM, mg	195	255
(685 mg/100 g cereal)		

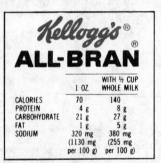

Kellogg's® ALL-BRAN®

	1 OZ.	WITH ½ CUP WHOLE MILK
CALORIES	70	140
PROTEIN	4 g	8 g
CARBOHYDRATE	21 g	27 g
FAT	1 g	5 g
SODIUM	320 mg (1130 mg per 100 g)	380 mg (255 mg per 100 g)

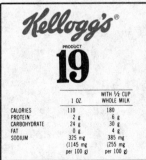

Kellogg's® PRODUCT 19

	1 OZ.	WITH ½ CUP WHOLE MILK
CALORIES	110	180
PROTEIN	2 g	6 g
CARBOHYDRATE	24 g	30 g
FAT	0 g	4 g
SODIUM	325 mg (1145 mg per 100 g)	385 mg (255 mg per 100 g)

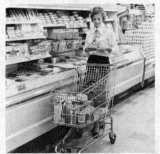

1

UNDERSTANDING HIGH BLOOD PRESSURE

A Symptom . . .
Not a
Disease

The doctors call it hypertension. You and I know it as high blood pressure.

Hypertension is a condition in which one has a higher blood pressure than judged to be normal.

Hypertension is not a disease . . . it is a symptom and its importance depends on the significance of its cause!

Organic hypertension is often due to diseases of the:

1. Heart and arteries
   (atherosclerosis, arteriosclerosis)[1]

2. Kidneys
   (glomerulonephritis)

3. Internal secretory glands

Organic hypertension is mostly acquired. Organic hypertension tends to progress . . . sometimes slow, sometimes quite rapidly. As the progress becomes more acute, it may strike a "target organ." It may strike the cerebral blood vessels, causing a

---

[1]Atherosclerosis: A form of arteriosclerosis in which there are localized accumulations of lipid-containing material within or beneath the inner coat of blood vessels.

Arteriosclerosis: A condition in which there is a thickening, hardening, and loss of elasticity of the walls of blood vessels, especially arteries.

stroke. It may hit the coronaries, causing a heart attack (myocardial infarction). It may effect the kidneys, causing uremia, or your eyes, causing blindness.

SIDE EFFECTS POSSIBLE

Drugs May Produce Adverse Effects

Most physicians try to use the least toxic drugs for mild hypertension.

The Medical Letter on Drugs and Therapeutics, a publication for doctors, states on page 23 of its January, 1975 issue:

All antihypertensive drugs can cause severe adverse effects.

On page 24 of the same newsletter:

Reserpine and other rauwolfia alkaloids deplete tissue of stores of catecholamines[1] and 5-hydroxytryptamine (serotonin), including those in the central nervous system. Their most disturbing adverse effect is psychic depression that can lead to suicide.

A history of depression is an absolute contraindication to use of rauwolfia alkaloids, but severe depression can also occur in patients without such a history when they take these drugs.

An increased incidence of breast cancer has been reported in patients treated with reserpine (Lancet, 2:669, 672, 675, 1974), although a cause-and-effect relationship has not been established.

[1]Catecholamines: Biologically active amines, epinephrine and norepinephrine, derived from the amino acid tyrosine. They have a marked effect on the nervous and cardiovascular systems, metabolic rate, temperature, and smooth muscle.

**No
Drug
Entirely
Safe**

It might be pointed out that The Medical Letter on Drugs and Therapeutics is an independent non-profit publication which provides unbiased critical evaluations of drugs in terms of their effectiveness, adverse effects, and possible alternative medications.

For treatment The Medical Letter continues, in part, on page 25:

> Drug treatment should start with a thiazide-type diuretic; if this does not produce an adequate response, a second drug may be needed.

From the previous quotations it should be observed that no drug is really entirely safe or completely adequate in the treating of high blood pressure.

Adrenalin
A secretion of the two small adrenal glands above the kidneys. The secretion, also called epinephrine, constricts the small blood vessels (arterioles), increases heart beat rate, and raises blood pressure.

Aneurysm
A sac-like bulging of the wall of an artery or vein, resulting from weakening of the wall by disease or present as an abnormality at birth.

Angina Pectoris
Chest pain caused by inadequate blood supply to the heart muscle, commonly the result of narrowing of the arteries feeding the heart muscle by atherosclerosis.

Anoxia
Lack of oxygen. Most often occurs when blood supply to a part of the body is completely cut off. This leads to death of the tissue.

Antihypertensive Agent
A drug used to lower blood pressure.

Aorta
The main trunk artery of the body. It begins at the base of the heart, receives blood from the heart's main pumping chamber (left ventricle). After arching up over the heart somewhat like the handle of a cane, it passes down through chest and abdomen in front of the spine. From the aorta, branch off many arteries that carry blood to all areas of the body except the lungs, which get blood through other vessels coming directly from the heart.

Apoplexy
Also called apoplectic stroke or stroke. A sudden shutoff of blood flow to a part of the brain as the result of blockage or rupture of an artery. It may first lead to loss of consciousness, sensation or voluntary movement, and may leave part of the body, often one side, temporarily or permanently paralyzed.

Arrhythmia
An abnormal heart beat rhythm.

Arterioles
The smallest arterial vessels (about 1/125 inch in diameter). They pass blood from arteries to capillaries, the latter being vessels through which oxygen and nutrients can move into the tissues.

Arteriosclerosis
Hardening of the arteries. A broad term that includes various conditions causing artery walls to thicken, harden, lose elasticity. See *Atherosclerosis.*

Artery
A blood vessel transporting blood away from the heart to a body area.

Atheroma
A deposit of materials, including fatty substances, in the inner lining of an artery wall, characteristic of atherosclerosis.

Atherosclerosis
A kind of arteriosclerosis in which the inner layer of the artery wall is made thick and irregular by deposits of fatty substances and other materials. The deposits, extending above the normal surface of the inner layer of the artery, decrease the diameter of the vessel's internal channel.

Calorie
A unit that expresses food energy. It represents the amount of heat needed to raise the temperature of 1 kilogram of water 1 degree centigrade. A high calorie diet has a caloric value above the total daily energy requirement; a low calorie diet has a caloric value below the energy requirement.

Capillaries
Very narrow tubes that form a network between arterioles and veins. Their walls consist of just a single layer of cells through which oxygen and nutrients pass to the tissues and carbon dioxide and waste products pass from tissues into blood stream.

Cardiovascular-Renal Disease
Disease involving heart, blood vessels, and kidneys.

Carotid Arteries
The left and right common carotid arteries are the principal vessels supplying the head and neck. Each has two major branches, external and internal carotid.

Cerebral Vascular Accident
Also called apoplectic stroke or stroke. A sudden interruption of blood supply to part of the brain.

Chemotherapy
The treatment of disease by use of chemicals. Thus, chemotherapy of hypertension is the treatment of high blood pressure by drugs.

Cholesterol
A fatlike substance found in animal tissue. In blood tests, the normal level for Americans is considered to be between 180 and 230 milligrams of cholesterol for each 100 cubic centimeters of blood.

Congestive Heart Failure
When the heart loses some of its efficiency and is unable to pump out all the blood that returns to it, blood backs up in the veins leading to the heart. Congestion, or fluid accumulation, in lungs, legs, abdomen, or other parts of the body may result from the heart's failure to maintain satisfactory circulation.

Coronary Arteries
The two arteries that branch off from the aorta and carry blood to the heart muscle.

Coronary Atherosclerosis
Commonly called coronary heart disease. A thickening by abnormal deposits of the inner layer of the walls of the coronary arteries carrying blood to the heart muscle. With the thickening, the internal channel of the arteries becomes narrowed and blood supply to the heart muscle is reduced.

Coronary Occlusion
An obstruction, usually a blood clot, in a branch of a coronary artery. The obstruction impedes blood flow to some part of the heart muscle that dies because of lack of nourishment. Sometimes called a coronary heart attack, or heart attack.

Coronary Thrombosis
The development of a clot in a coronary artery branch. A form of coronary occlusion. See *Coronary Occlusion.*

Diuretic
A drug that promotes excretion of urine.

Dyspnea
Difficult or labored breathing.

Edema
Swelling due to abnormal amounts of fluid retained in the body tissues.

Embolism
The obstruction of a blood vessel by a clot or other material carried in the blood stream from another site.

Essential Hypertension
Commonly known as high blood pressure; sometimes called primary hypertension; an elevated pressure not caused by kidney or other evident disease.

Hemiplegia
Paralysis of one side of the body as the result of damage to the opposite side of the brain. Nerves cross in the brain so that one side of the brain controls the opposite arm and leg. Such paralysis is sometimes caused by a blood clot or hemorrhage in a brain blood vessel. See Stroke.

Hypertension
Commonly called high blood pressure. May be *essential* hypertension, without known cause, or *secondary* hypertension, stemming from kidney or other disease.

Hypotension
Commonly called low blood pressure. Blood pressure below the normal range.

Infarct
An area of tissue damaged or dead as a result of receiving insufficient blood. As used in the phrase "myocardial infarct" it refers to a heart muscle area damaged or killed by insufficient blood flow through a coronary artery that normally supplies the area.

Ischemia
A localized and usually temporary shortage of blood in some part of the body that may be caused by a constriction or obstruction in a blood vessel supplying that part.

Lipid
Fat.

Metabolism
All the chemical changes that take place within the body.

Myocardial Infarction
Damage or death of an area of the heart muscle (myocardium) caused by reduced blood supply reaching the area.

Nitroglycerin
A vasodilator drug that relaxes the muscles in blood vessels. Often used to relieve or help prevent attacks of angina pectoris.

Primary Hypertension
Also called essential hypertension and commonly known as high blood pressure. An elevated pressure not related to kidney or other apparent disease.

Psychosomatic
Having to do with the influence of mind and emotions upon the functions of the body, especially in terms of disease.

Renal Hypertension
High blood pressure caused by damage to or disease of the kidneys.

Sclerosis
Hardening, usually due to accumulation of fibrous material.

Secondary Hypertension
Elevated blood pressure caused by — therefore, secondary to — a specific disease.

Sphygmomanometer
An instrument for measuring blood pressure in the arteries.

Stroke
Also called apoplectic stroke, cerebrovascular accident, or cerebral vascular accident. The result of impeded blood supply to some part of the brain that may be caused by **(1)** a blood clot forming in the vessel wall (cerebral thrombosis); **(2)** a rupture of a blood vessel wall and escape of blood into the brain area nearby (cerebral hemorrhage); **(3)** a clot or other material from elsewhere in the circulatory system that flows to the brain and obstructs a brain vessel (cerebral embolism); **(4)** pressure on a blood vessel, as by a tumor.

Toxemia
The condition produced by poisonous substances in the blood.

Uremia
Excess in the blood of waste materials normally excreted by the kidneys in the urine.

Vasoconstrictor
Vasoconstrictor nerves are those in the involuntary, or autonomic system which, when stimulated, cause arteriole muscles to contract, thus narrowing the arterioles, increasing their resistance to blood flow, and raising blood pressure. Chemical substances that contract the arteriole muscles are called vasoconstrictor agents, or vasopressors. One example is adrenalin, or epinephrine.

Vasodilator
Vasodilator nerves are those in the involuntary, or autonomic system which, when stimulated, cause arteriole muscles to relax, enlarging the arteriole passage, reducing resistance to blood flow, and lowering blood pressure. Vasodilator agents are chemicals that cause relaxation of arteriole muscles. Nitroglycerin is one example.

Vaso-Inhibitor
A drug that inhibits action of the vasomotor nerves and thus causes arteriole muscles to relax, the arteriole passage to enlarge, and blood pressure to be lowered.

Vasopressor
A drug that contracts muscles of the arterioles, narrowing the arteriole passage and raising blood pressure. Such a substance also is called a vasoconstrictor. One example is adrenalin, or epinephrine.

Vein
A vessel that carries blood from a part of the body back to the heart. All veins conduct unoxygenated, or used blood, except the pulmonary veins, which carry freshly oxygenated blood from the lungs back to the heart.

STRESS ENCOURAGES HYPERTENSION

AN OBSESSION FOR POSSESSIONS

We Live in a STRESS Environment

We are living in an age of STRESS! Advertisers on television have conditioned most people that they simply cannot live or enjoy life without their product. **Therefore the grand race begins of trying to earn enough money to buy "just one more thing."**

Then, on the other hand, ravaging inflation sometimes makes it necessary for one to hold two jobs just to be able to feed his family and provide them with essential clothes and pay the mortgage.

And to this add the "quickie" meals at fast-food fare drive-ins . . . with their fat-saturated hamburgers and heart-attack inducing french fries.

And what do you come up with?

STRESS!

And what can stress lead to?

HIGH BLOOD PRESSURE plus a myriad other ills!

THE DANGERS OF STRESS

Warning Signs

So to stay fresh and awake . . . when we get run-down, we gulp a cup of coffee.

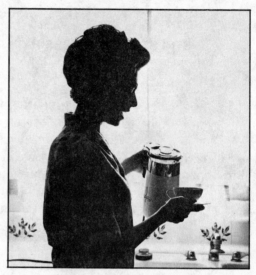

Soon we notice warning signs of improper living:

1. *Frequent headaches*
2. *Inner discontent*
3. *Restlessness*
4. *Weak concentration*
5. *Mild agitation*
6. *Loss of sense of humor*

Work, which previously satisfied us now becomes a painful burden.

In the second stage, we notice anxious sensations of heart pain and nervous outbreaks of perspiring.

At the third stage we discover we have high blood pressure or suffer a stroke, a nervous breakdown or experience a heart attack.

When it reaches this point, the breakdown in our health may be so severe that a complete recovery is not possible.

An Ounce of Prevention

The purpose of this book is primarily to make you aware of proper health maintenance before an irreversible illness occurs. I need not remind you that "an ounce of prevention is worth a pound of cure!" But I'll remind you anyway!

An ounce of prevention
IS (there is no doubt about it)
worth
a pound of cure!

In hypertension—high blood pressure—a variety of factors from malfunction to nervous strain may combine to create a resistance to the flow of blood through the arterioles, causing the heart to pump harder to surmount this obstacle.

WISE ADVICE FROM THE BIBLE

The Sins of our Fathers

The Bible, in Numbers 14:18 says:

> *The Lord is long-suffering,*
>   *and of great mercy,*
> *forgiving iniquity and transgression,*
>   *and by no means clearing the guilty,*
>   *visiting the iniquity of the fathers*
>   *upon the children*
>   *unto the third and fourth generation.*

AVOID THESE FOODS

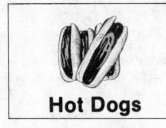

Hot Dogs

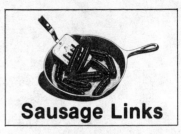

Sausage Links

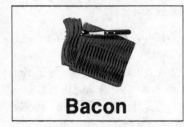

Bacon

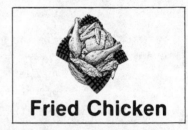

Fried Chicken

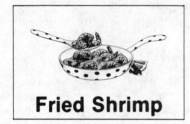

Fried Shrimp

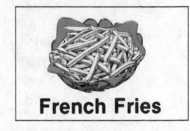

French Fries

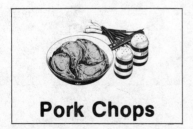

Pork Chops

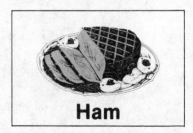

Ham

**Our Body
A Temple**

In the New Testament in 1 Corinthians 3:16,17 we read:

> *Know ye not
>   that ye are the temple of God . . .
> If any man defile the temple of God,
>   him shall God destroy;
>   for the temple of God is holy,
>   which temple ye are.*

This is further emphasized in 1 Corinthians 6:19 which states:

> *Know ye not
>   that your body
> is the temple of the Holy Ghost . . .*

**Don't
Make It
A
Garbage
Dump!**

If our body, created by God, is God's temple, then, what we eat is important. And if we defile that temple by eating foods that are detrimental to health . . . by smoking, by drinking . . . then God says he will **destroy** that one who treats God's holy temple in an unholy way.

In the Old Testament verse in Numbers, which we previously quoted, we are told that the Lord is long-suffering. And indeed diseases caused by High Blood Pressure usually do not appear until after 35.

Do people inherit High Blood Pressure? NO! But if there is a history of High Blood Pressure in your family . . . the chances are you may inherit poor eating habits. And it is these sins which are passed on . . . *unto the third and fourth generation."*

3

HEALTHY ARTERIES THE KEY

SMALL BUT VITAL

How's Your Arterial Resiliency?

Arterioles are minute arteries. The heart of a man with hypertension may fill half his chest cavity.

In arterial disease the arteries lose their resiliency, the walls harden as a result of the deposit of fatty materials and calcium.

Healthy arterial walls, however, stretch and rebound with each heartbeat.

Fasting aids in the purification of these arteries. Toxics are flushed out of the body, unneeded fat is "burned up" and excreted.

One starts to feel young again, there is a lightness in the body, an alertness in the mind.

Fasting, combined with sensible eating habits, is beneficial in the lowering of one's blood pressure.

The arteries of the heart are small. The largest arteries in the heart are no wider than a thin soda straw.

There is much truth in the saying:

You are as old as your arteries.

NORMAL HEART

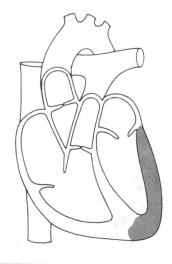

HYPERTENSIVE HEART
Red area indicates thickening of the wall of the ventricle. This is a reaction of the heart to high blood pressure.

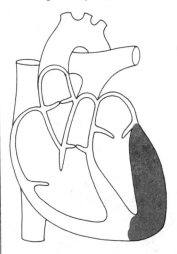

NORMAL KIDNEY

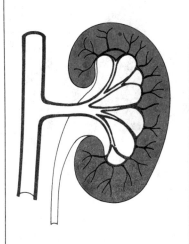

HYPERTENSIVE KIDNEY

(1) Fiberplasia (over-growth of tissue) interferes with blood flow.

(2) Note how the small arteries of the kidney are narrower and constricted. This narrowing is artherosclerosis.

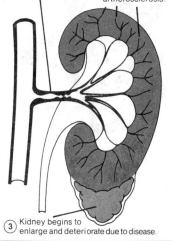

(3) Kidney begins to enlarge and deteriorate due to disease.

**The
Silent
Killer**

Heart disease is the number one cause of death among all Americans over the age of 35. Strokes rank third as a cause of death. To a large extent, both of these diseases are caused by High Blood Pressure, as well as kidney failure.

High Blood Pressure is often referred to as the *"silent killer"* because it rarely produces warning signals.

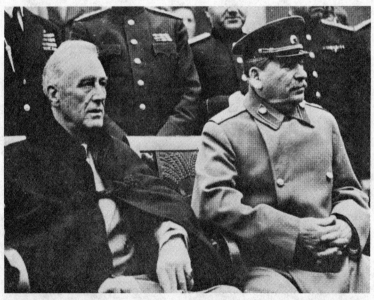

At the Yalta Conference in 1945 both Franklin Roosevelt and Joseph Stalin suffered from high blood pressure (hypertension). Later, both died of strokes . . . Roosevelt in April, 1945 and Stalin in 1953.

4

WHAT IS BLOOD PRESSURE?

WHAT IS BLOOD PRESSURE?

Persistent Pressure Dangerous

The adult human body has some 60,000 miles of blood vessels. As the body's blood (5 quarts or more in the average adult) is pumped by the heart through arteries, capillaries and veins, it exerts force on the walls of these vessels. Like pipes in a plumbing system, the arteries can tolerate high pressure for brief surges. But persistent pressure is dangerous. One out of every four Americans is affected with High Blood Pressure.

The only way medically to define whether you have High Blood Pressure is by having a doctor check your blood pressure. After age 40, adults should have their blood pressure checked annually.

SOME POPULAR MISCONCEPTIONS

A Middle Age Disease

It is often said that blood pressure should normally measure *"100 plus your age,"* and that *"low blood pressure"* is a dangerous condition. Neither of these notions is true. People do tend to develop High Blood Pressure as they approach middle age, es-

SYSTOLIC PRESSURE is the peak of pressure when the heart contracts (beats) to force blood out into the arteries. Pressure is measured by the rise of a column of mercury on a blood pressure instrument that includes an inflatable rubber cuff (sphygmomanometer).

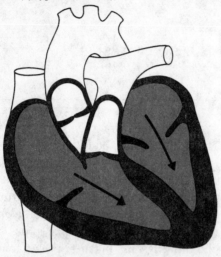

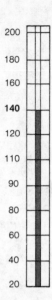

DIASTOLIC PRESSURE is a measurement of the constant minimum pressure when the heart relaxes between beats and fills its chambers.

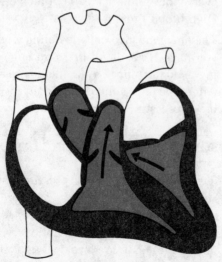

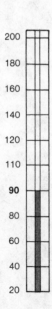

pecially harried businessmen and nerve-racked housewives, but there is no rule-of-thumb increase in normal blood pressure according to age. A blood pressure of 140/100 is just as abnormal for a man of 65 as it is for a girl of 18.[1]

NORMAL BLOOD PRESSURE

Average Blood Pressure

The average normal reading for blood pressure is:

$\underline{120}$ systolic
80   diastolic

This means that when the heart contracts (goes into "*systole*") and squeezes blood out into the arteries, the pressure in the arteries rises to 120 millimeters of mercury.

When your heart relaxes (goes into "*diastole*"), the pressure in the arteries drops to 80 millimeters of mercury.

The walls of the arteries are able to tolerate these pressures without any difficulty.

In blood pressure readings, the lower figure (*diastolic level*) is the more accurate indicator of blood-pressure disease.[2]

---

[1]Alan E. Nourse, M.D., Ladies' Home Journal Family Medical Guide, (New York: Harper & Row, Publishers), 1973, p. 584.

[2]*Diastolic pressure* is the point of least pressure in the arterial vascular system. When the diastolic pressure fails to drop in proportion to the systolic pressure, this is a danger sign.

HIGH BLOOD PRESSURE FIGURES

Several Readings Required

High Blood Pressure (*Hypertension*) is when one's blood pressure is consistently higher than

<u>140</u> systolic
90 diastolic

One reading taken at a doctor's office or for an insurance examination is not sufficient to diagnose an individual as having High Blood Pressure. Your pressure may be up due to nervousness. Accurate readings should be taken over 2 or 3 day periods.

Women tolerate High Blood Pressure better than men. Those who smoke and those who have diabetes are more susceptible to High Blood Pressure and greater arterial damage.

Hyper (as in Hypertension) means that the blood pressure is higher than normal.

The term "*malignant hypertension*" refers to a type of High Blood Pressure that is unusually severe. It has nothing to do with cancer.

Some recent medical tests in 1981 seem to indicate that people with a high systolic reading (the top figure) have twice as many strokes as those with normal blood pressures . . . regardless of their diastolic pressure (lower figure) levels. This new report comes from the Journal of the American Medical Association.

5

WHAT CAUSES HIGH BLOOD PRESSURE?

WHAT CAUSES HIGH BLOOD PRESSURE?

Hardening of Arteries

Hardening of the arteries is the greatest single factor in the development of High Blood Pressure. This is called **arteriosclerosis.** The arteries become narrower and less elastic and the heart must pump harder to get blood to circulate through them. It is the forceful contraction of the heart that is recorded as High Blood Pressure.[1]

Hardening of the arteries in the kidneys (renal artery) is one of the commonest causes of high blood pressure.

People do not inherit High Blood Pressure. In general doctors do not know exactly what causes High Blood Pressure. They suggest that contributory conditions include being overweight (obesity), excessive cigarette smoking and excessive intake of salt with meals. They do not accept the premise that diet is related to High Blood Pressure. Yet, if High Blood Pressure appears to run in certain families . . . nutritionists would assume that diet is indeed the culprit.

[1]Robert E. Rothenberg, M.D., Health In The Later Years, (New York: New American Library), 1964, p. 358.

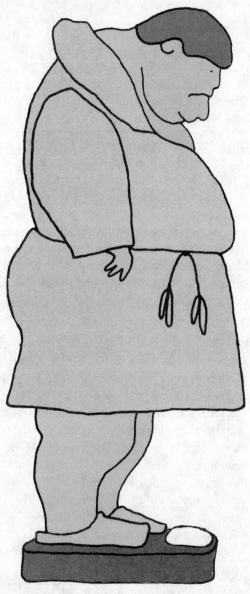

´i wonder
if it was the
maraschino
cherry?´

(Illustration courtesy LIFE & HEALTH)

TWO CAUSES REVEALED

Too Much Salt!

The Harvard Medical School Health Letter reports on two factors that encourage High Blood Pressure:

1. Salt Intake

... human societies in which individual daily salt intake averages less than 4 grams (about 2 teaspoons)

versus

the average American consumption of 12 grams (about 6 teaspoons) show a greatly reduced occurence
of hypertension.

... the hidden salt in the processed food of the typical American diet is a real hazard.

One ounce of Corn Flakes contains twice as much sodium as an equivalent serving of Planters Peanuts, and a Big Mac comes loaded with five times as much sodium as the one ounce serving of Corn Flakes.

Too Much Weight

2. Excessive Weight

Many studies have now documented that obesity increases the risk of hypertension
...

It has been demonstrated that weight loss can serve as effective treatment for high blood pressure—
and is sometimes all that's needed in mild cases.[1]

[1]G. Timothy Johnson, M.D., A Look At High Blood Pressure—Part II, (Cambridge, Mass., Harvard Medical School), July, 1979, Vol. IV, Number 9, page 1.

6

HYPERTENSION CAN CAUSE SERIOUS ILLNESS

TWO TYPES OF HYPERTENSION

**Primary
Hypertension
Most
Frequent**

Hypertension is classified as primary and secondary.

Primary hypertension covers the majority of cases of High Blood Pressure and refers to hypertension that has no easily identifiable and remediable cause.

**Secondary
Hypertension
Can Be
Corrected**

Secondary hypertension is High Blood Pressure that has an identifiable and correctable underlying cause—such as a narrowed artery leading to a kidney or an adrenal gland tumor.[1] These cases are less frequent and can be corrected by surgery.

POSSIBLE WARNING SIGNS

**Morning
Headaches**

As we said previously, High Blood Pressure does not display any usual symp-

---

[1]*Pheochromocytoma* is a non-cancerous adrenal gland tumor than can be surgically removed.

toms. Some people, when told they have High Blood Pressure, relate that they suffer from "*morning headaches,*" a dull aching pain in the back of the head that is present upon arising but disappears once the person is up and about.

Other Symptoms

Other symptoms may include dizziness, excessive nervous irritability or even vomiting.

AFFECTS THREE AREAS

If blood pressure is allowed to climb abnormally high without treatment or control, three areas of the body can be affected

1. **Heart**

   Enlargement of the heart as the muscle walls thicken in an effort to handle the extra load. Finally this will cause *congestive heart failure.* Furthermore, small arterioles and capillaries all over the body can break and hemorrhage because of this continuing pressure. Vision can be affected.

2. **Cerebral Hemorrhage**

   The bursting of a blood vessel in the brain can cause a stroke (CVA or *cerebrovascular accident*). Sometimes such a stroke may only cause minor damage. However, if the condition is not corrected a stroke will occur large enough to cause death.

3. Uremia

Uremia
Greatest
Danger

The greatest number of deaths from High Blood Pressure is that condition known as uremia. The individual, initially, has a gradual loss of kidney function resulting in damage to the tiny arterioles in the kidneys over a period of years. Uremia is when the kidneys finally cease to function at all. The kidneys fail to filter out nitrogen-containing waste products. The poisonous chemicals begin piling up in the blood stream. Blood may even seep into the urine, from the kidneys.

High Blood Pressure is a contributing factor to atherosclerosis, coronary artery disease and coronary thrombosis.

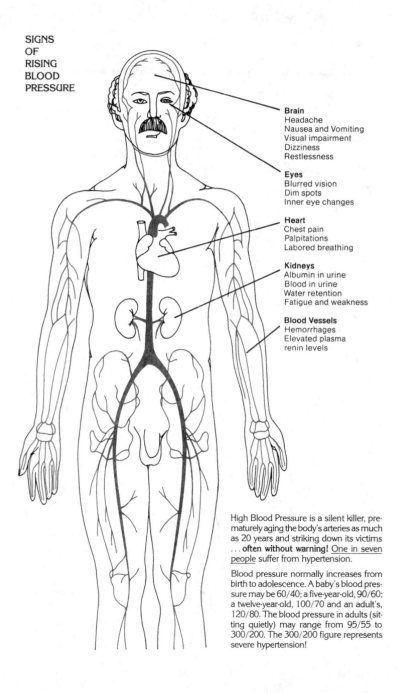

SIGNS OF RISING BLOOD PRESSURE

Brain
Headache
Nausea and Vomiting
Visual impairment
Dizziness
Restlessness

Eyes
Blurred vision
Dim spots
Inner eye changes

Heart
Chest pain
Palpitations
Labored breathing

Kidneys
Albumin in urine
Blood in urine
Water retention
Fatigue and weakness

Blood Vessels
Hemorrhages
Elevated plasma
renin levels

High Blood Pressure is a silent killer, prematurely aging the body's arteries as much as 20 years and striking down its victims . . . **often without warning!** One in seven people suffer from hypertension.

Blood pressure normally increases from birth to adolescence. A baby's blood pressure may be 60/40; a five-year-old, 90/60; a twelve-year-old, 100/70 and an adult's, 120/80. The blood pressure in adults (sitting quietly) may range from 95/55 to 300/200. The 300/200 figure represents severe hypertension!

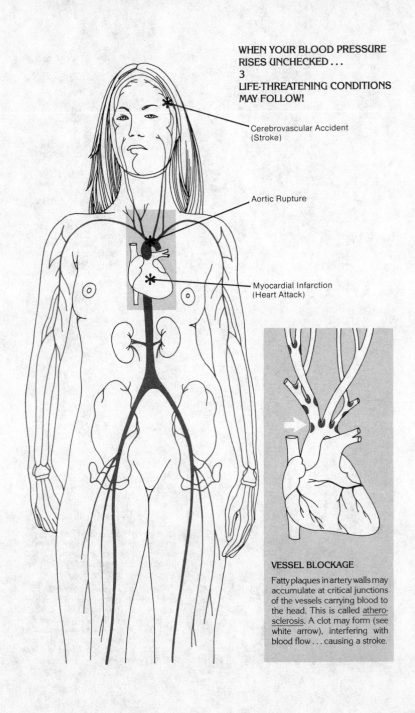

WHEN YOUR BLOOD PRESSURE
RISES UNCHECKED ...
3
LIFE-THREATENING CONDITIONS
MAY FOLLOW!

Cerebrovascular Accident
(Stroke)

Aortic Rupture

Myocardial Infarction
(Heart Attack)

VESSEL BLOCKAGE

Fatty plaques in artery walls may accumulate at critical junctions of the vessels carrying blood to the head. This is called athero-sclerosis. A clot may form (see white arrow), interfering with blood flow ... causing a stroke.

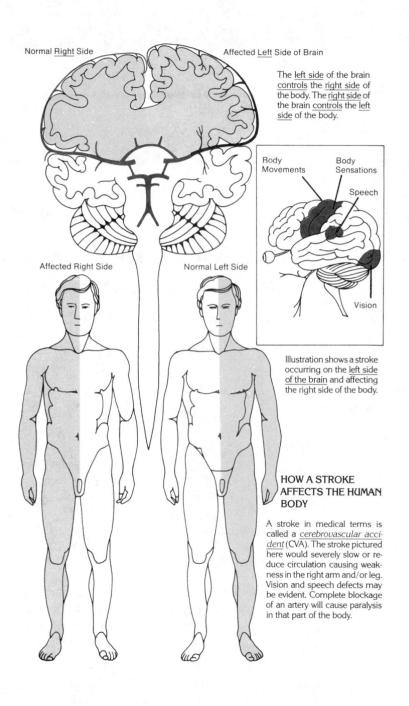

Normal <u>Right</u> Side

Affected <u>Left</u> Side of Brain

The <u>left side</u> of the brain <u>controls</u> the <u>right side</u> of the body. The <u>right side</u> of the brain <u>controls</u> the <u>left side</u> of the body.

Body Movements

Body Sensations

Speech

Vision

Affected Right Side

Normal Left Side

Illustration shows a stroke occurring on the <u>left side of the brain</u> and affecting the right side of the body.

HOW A STROKE AFFECTS THE HUMAN BODY

A stroke in medical terms is called a <u>*cerebrovascular accident*</u> (CVA). The stroke pictured here would severely slow or reduce circulation causing weakness in the right arm and/or leg. Vision and speech defects may be evident. Complete blockage of an artery will cause paralysis in that part of the body.

7

THE MEDICAL APPROACH
TO
HIGH BLOOD PRESSURE

Drug Therapy
Usual
Medical
Treatment

Medical treatment for High Blood Pressure falls into three categories:

1. **Life Style Changes**
   Restrictions are put on salt intake and, if a person is obese, weight loss is recommended.

2. **Behavioral Therapies**
   Persons with constant drive are shown the art of relaxation, meditation and biofeedback.

3. **Drug Therapy**
   If blood pressure reading is above 160/100 one or more drugs will be used to bring pressure levels into normal range.

By far, drug therapy is the primary approach medically to High Blood Pressure. Outside of the suggestion that you reduce your salt intake ... not much nutritional advice is given.

FOUR MAJOR DRUG GROUPS

**Prevents
Sodium
Build-up!**

1. Diuretics *("Fluid pills")*
The exact reasons for the effectiveness of these drugs, which promote increased urinary excretion of sodium, are not known.[1] Diuretics reduce blood volume by causing the excretion of fluid through the kidneys. Their main use in treating hypertension is to prevent the sodium and water retention caused by other drugs.

**Widens
Blood
Vessels**

2. Direct-Acting Vasodilators
These drugs widen blood vessels by acting on them directly. They are usually combined with diuretics and side effects may occur. All vasodilators produce varying degrees of sodium and water retention. That is why diuretics are given at the same time.

**Acts
As
Regulator**

3. Sympathetic Inhibitors
These drugs modify nervous system control of blood vessels in a manner that allows the vessels to dilate and thus decrease pressure. To *dilate* means to make wider or larger. The word *sympathetic* refers to the sym-

[1]G. Timothy Johnson, M.D., A Look At High Blood Pressure—Part II (Cambridge, Mass., Harvard Medical School), July, 1979, Vol. IV, Number 9, page 2.

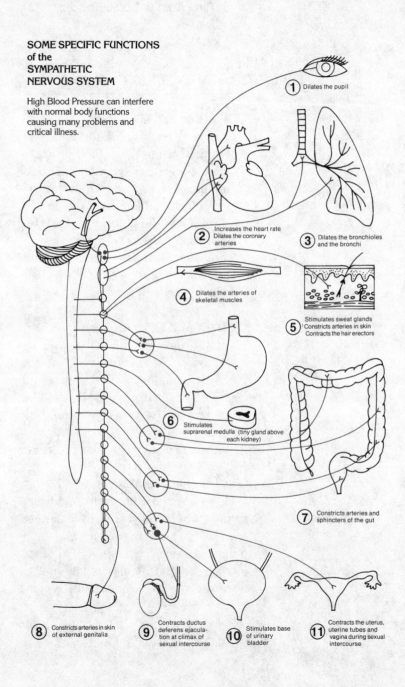

SOME SPECIFIC FUNCTIONS
of the
SYMPATHETIC
NERVOUS SYSTEM

High Blood Pressure can interfere with normal body functions causing many problems and critical illness.

1 Dilates the pupil

2 Increases the heart rate
Dilates the coronary arteries

3 Dilates the bronchioles and the bronchi

4 Dilates the arteries of skeletal muscles

5 Stimulates sweat glands
Constricts arteries in skin
Contracts the hair erectors

6 Stimulates suprarenal medulla (tiny gland above each kidney)

7 Constricts arteries and sphincters of the gut

8 Constricts arteries in skin of external genitalia

9 Contracts ductus deferens ejaculation at climax of sexual intercourse

10 Stimulates base of urinary bladder

11 Contracts the uterus, uterine tubes and vagina during sexual intercourse

The SYMPATHETIC Nervous System

The Sympathetic nervous system is part of the <u>autonomic</u> (involuntary) nervous system. It regulates functions at the unconscious level to control <u>involuntary</u> body functions. Such involuntary body functions would include: heart function, respiration and digestion.

The <u>Sympathetic</u> nervous system work in an <u>opposite</u> pattern to the <u>Parasympathetic</u> nervous system. As an example:

<u>The Sympathetic nervous system</u>
    releases at their nerve endings . . . <u>noradrenaline</u>
    This brings about
        <u>relaxation</u> of the muscle in the intestinal wall and
        <u>constriction</u> of the rings of the muscle (sphincters)
            such as found at the exit from the stomach.

<u>The Parasympathetic nervous system</u>
    releases at their nerve endings . . . <u>acetylcholine</u>
    This brings about
        <u>contraction</u> of the muscle of the intestinal wall and
        <u>relaxation</u> of the rings of the muscle (sphincters).

The <u>Sympathetic</u> nervous system goes to practically every part of the body. The <u>Parasympathetic</u> nervous system supply principally the stomach area. Para means *"on either side of"* and the Parasympathetic nerves emerge from the brain on either side of the Sympathetic nerves.

In the Sympathetic nervous system, the nerve fibers when stimulated release epinephrine (adrenaline) at their endings. The medical term for this is <u>adrenergic.</u> (The sweat glands, however, release <u>acetylcholine</u> and the medical term for this is <u>cholinergic</u>).

The Sympathetic nervous system is divided into **two** main parts:

<u>Alpha-adrenergic component</u>
    Comprises the vasoconstrictor nerves
        which causes blood vessels to constrict;
        that is, to become narrow.

<u>Beta-adrenergic component</u>
    Comprises the heart-stimulating nerves and
    the lung dilating nerves as well as the
    vasodilator nerves in voluntary muscle

The Sympathetic and Parasympathetic nervous system control the tiny arterioles. The arterioles relax and constrict affecting blood pressure. That is why hypertensive drugs are often prescribed to guide the action of the Sympathetic nervous system. These drugs reset blood pressue control mechanisms to acceptable limits.

pathetic nervous system, a part of the nervous system that is concerned with control of involuntary bodily functions of glands, smooth muscle tissue and the heart. It is this system which regulates increased heart rate and blood pressure.

Reduces
Heart
Output

4. Ganglionic Blocker

The ganglion is a mass of nervous tissue composed principally of nerve-cell bodies and lying outside the brain or spinal cord. These drugs (ganglionic blockers) block the point of contact between adjacent neurons, where nerve impulses are transmitted from one to the other. Blocking these contacts causes dilation (widening) of both arterioles (small, minute arteries) and veins. This results in lowered blood pressure and reduced heart output.

TREATMENTS BEGIN WITH DIURETIC

Results
Start
In
Four Days

Drug treatments usually begin with a thiazide-type diuretic which generally lowers blood pressure within three or four days. The reduction is usually moderate. Such drugs include (in the benzthiazide family) Aquapres, Aqua-Scrip, Aquasec, Aquastat, Aquatag, Directic, Diucen, Exna, Hydrex, Lemazide, Marazide, Proaqua, Rid-ema, S-Aqua and Urazide.

Tranquilizers Described

Half of the patients with mild hypertension only require a diuretic (thiazide or chlorthalidone). When additional therapy is needed, the second drug given is usually methyldopa or hydralazine. Trade names for methyldopa include: Aldomet, Dopamet, Medimet and Novomedopa. Trade names for hydralazine include: Apresoline, Dralzine, Hydralyn, Nor-Pres 25, Rolazine.

In addition to drugs given directly for the treatment of High Blood Pressure, sometimes a tranquilizer is prescribed to reduce stress conditions the patient may be under. Among the most common are Librium and Valium.

Although drugs such as Valium act quicker one must also consider the serious side effects.

An Alternative

As an alternative, some nutritionists suggest nature's tranquilizer. It is an amino acid called Tryptophan.

In a report in the British medical journal, Lancet (November 8, 1975, p. 920), the amino acid Tryptophan was shown to be as beneficial as a drug tranquilizer with fewer side effects.

Site and Action of Major Blood Pressure Drugs

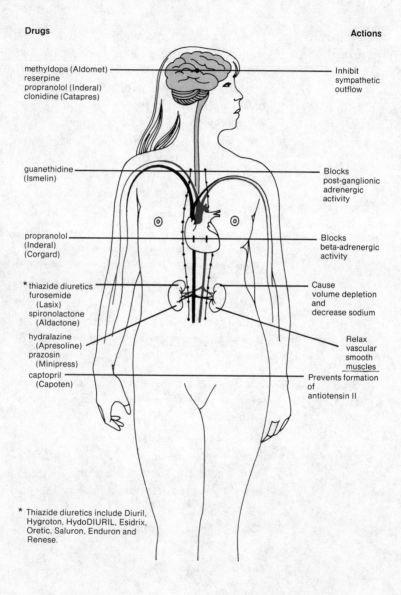

Drugs

methyldopa (Aldomet)
reserpine
propranolol (Inderal)
clonidine (Catapres)

guanethidine
(Ismelin)

propranolol
(Inderal)
(Corgard)

* thiazide diuretics
furosemide
(Lasix)
spironolactone
(Aldactone)

hydralazine
(Apresoline)
prazosin
(Minipress)
captopril
(Capoten)

Actions

Inhibit
sympathetic
outflow

Blocks
post-ganglionic
adrenergic
activity

Blocks
beta-adrenergic
activity

Cause
volume depletion
and
decrease sodium

Relax
vascular
smooth
muscles
Prevents formation
of
antiotensin II

* Thiazide diuretics include Diuril,
Hygroton, HydoDIURIL, Esidrix,
Oretic, Saluron, Enduron and
Renese.

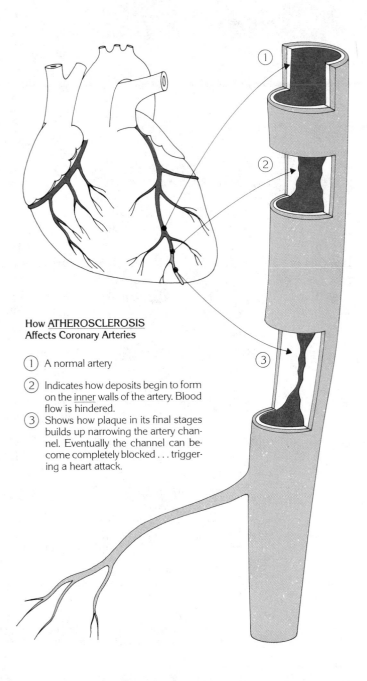

How <u>ATHEROSCLEROSIS</u>
Affects Coronary Arteries

(1) A normal artery

(2) Indicates how deposits begin to form
on the <u>inner</u> walls of the artery. Blood
flow is hindered.

(3) Shows how plaque in its final stages
builds up narrowing the artery channel. Eventually the channel can become completely blocked . . . trigger-
ing a heart attack.

8

THE NUTRITIONAL APPROACH
TO
HIGH BLOOD PRESSURE

**The Pritikin
And
Rinse Diets**

Many of the nutritional approaches to Heart Disease would be identical to the nutritional approaches to High Blood Pressure. For that reason, they are not listed here but will be found in the book, HEART DISEASE by Salem Kirban.[1]

The Pritikin Diet is a month-long program that is extremely low in fat, cholesterol, protein and refined carbohydrates. It is HIGH in complex carbohydrates, fruits and vegetables.[2] Pritikin has Longevity Centers in Santa Monica, California and Miami, Florida. The 26-day stay averages about $5500.

---

[1]**For a copy of HEART DISEASE by Salem Kirban,** send $5 (plus $1 for postage) to: Salem Kirban, Inc., Kent Road, Huntingdon Valley, Pennsylvania 19006.

[2]Complex Carbohydrates *(like lima beans or other vegetables and grains)* provide energy but do not raise blood fats.

Simple Carbohydrates *(like cupcakes, cakes, candy and other products with refined sugar)* will raise your blood fats and add weight. Sucrose is a simple carbohydrate.

The Rinse Diet was formulated by Jacobus Rinse, Ph.D. when his life was threatened by atherosclerosis. Atherosclerosis is a thickening and loss of elasticity in the inner walls of the arteries. From a layman's viewpoint, **arterio**sclerosis and **athero**sclerosis generally mean *"hardening of the arteries."* Jacobus Rinse put together a *"breakfast mash"* which included lecithin, sunflower seeds, bonemeal and about 7 other ingredients. Taking two tablespoons of this daily over his breakfast cereal or with juice, his heart problems did not recur and his energy level increased.

Both the Pritikin Diet and the Rinse Diet are described in detail in the book, **HEART DISEASE** by Salem Kirban.

Guidelines Similar

Because High Blood Pressure problems are so closely related with Heart Disease, strokes *(cerebrovascular accident/*CVA) and Diabetes . . . many of the medical approaches are similar. Also, nutritional guidelines for all 3 diseases follow similar patterns.

The Rinse Diet

Jacobus Rinse, Ph.D., discovered at the age of 51, that his life was threatened by atherosclerosis. He was troubled by repeated attacks of angina.

Rinse did not smoke. He was not overweight. His family had no incidence of heart disease. Nor did he eat creamy sauces or desserts. He searched scientific journals and came up with the conclusion that perhaps he had a nutritional deficiency.

He decided to put together a combination of ingredients that he hoped would correct the problem. He called it his *"breakfast mash."* He developed this formula after 7 years of trial and error and two serious heart attacks. It was in 1951 that his doctor gave him at the most, 10 years to live. This report is written in 1981 (30 years later) and Dr. Jacobus Rinse is still alive!

Dr. Rinse mixes with juice or other liquid:

> 5 grams of lecithin
> 12 grams of coarsely chopped sunflower seeds
> 5 grams of debittered Brewer's yeast
> 2 grams of bonemeal (dicalcium phosphate)
> 5 grams of raw wheat germ

With this he also takes:

> 500 milligrams Vitamin C
> 100 I.U. Vitamin E
> 40 milligrams Vitamin B_6 plus magnesium oxide and zinc supplements

Dr. Rinse reports that not only has he been free from the recurrence of his heart problems but his energy level has increased!

9

GARLIC . . . THE POOR MAN'S RICHES

A Medicine Used by Egyptians

If I had to choose between gold and garlic, I'd choose GARLIC . . . for it is nature's gold . . . and is one of nature's answers to High Blood Pressure!

Sophisticated people tend to shy away from it . . . for it has a pungent aroma that broadcasts without a radio!

Pets apparently love it and thrive on it . . . for most brands of pet food contain garlic.

Actually garlic comes from a well-bred line. It is part of the lily family, a cousin. But there is always one black sheep in the family.

For thousands of years garlic has been accepted as both a food and a medicine. The Egyptians had at least 22 therapeutic formulas using garlic about 2000 B.C. It was used for headaches, heart problems, body weakness, worms, problems of childbirth. The Egyptians even used it in their enemas! To them garlic was a god!

The Israelites had a hard time in Egypt. They were slaves and most were assigned to brickmaking. Pharoah made the task of brickmaking as difficult as possible. He

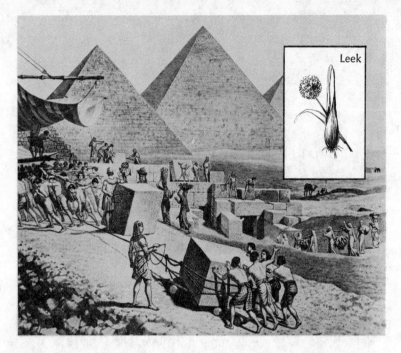

Leek

Garlic is only mentioned once in the Bible. After Moses had successfully guided the Israelites to safety from Pharaoh, they still yearned for the "... leeks and the onions and the garlic" of Egypt (Numbers 11:5). Their memories were short. They apparently forgot about the oppression of slavery that was their lot under Pharaoh.

Charcoal roasted whole garlic is still a Middle Eastern specialty. Place whole bulbs of garlic directly on the coals of a grille (but not in flaming fire). The cloves are ready when they are browned and tender. If you wish, you can marinate beforehand. You can baste the garlic heads with oil and herb seasonings after you remove from fire. The meat can be easily pushed out of the hardened skin. An excellent nutlike flavor. Garlic is rich in phosphorus and potassium. It has a high sulphur content. Sulphur has been termed the "beauty mineral" and is vital for healthy hair, skin and nails.

The leek (pictured in inset) resembles an onion. Leeks are very high in potassium and are excellent to use in soups.

did not supply the necessary straw for the bricks. The Israelites had to go search for it wherever they could find it. Hebrew officers were assigned to make sure the job got done. When quotas were not fulfilled, it was the Hebrew overseer who suffered.

From Suffering

He was made to lie on his stomach with his legs and feet upward. He would be struck many blows on the soles of his feet. This made it impossible for him to walk for weeks.

The Israelites began to murmur against Moses and Aaron, blaming them for Pharoah's oppressive attitude.

When Moses finally did lead the some 6 million Israelites out of Egypt, through the Red Sea and into the wilderness, the people still were not satisfied.

A LONGING FOR GARLIC

To Murmuring

All along the way they were complaining. Somehow they seemed to forget the unbearable demands of Pharoah and longed for the peasant food that they had once relished. And they complained to Moses:

> We remember the fish, which we did eat in Egypt freely; the cucumbers and the melons, and the leeks, and the onions and the garlic.
>
> (Numbers 11:5)

For Stress

Moses was at the end of his rope. He had had it with the complaints of the Israelites and in Numbers 11:15 went so far as to ask

God to kill him and release him from this continual round of complaints heaped upon him by his people. Even Moses was human and the pressure was getting to him. In those days there was no Vitamin B complex capsules and Vitamin C chewables to relieve his stress. But he could have eaten the garlic!

Wherever the Israelites had a garden, you could count on it containing garlic, onions and leeks.

10

GARLIC . . . THE REVITALIZER

FOR A HAPPIER LOVE LIFE!

**Garlic
A
Marital Aid**

The people of Israel believed that garlic, considered a "hot" food, had generative powers that gave the body life and marital energy.

The Talmund suggested the eating of garlic for gynecological and menstrual disturbances. Even in Russia and Poland today, Jews break their fast on bread and raw garlic.

Garlic, in fact, has a long history . . . going back much further than the times of Egyptian oppression of the people of Israel. The Chinese have used garlic for centuries.

UNUSUAL QUALITIES

**A
Healing
Food**

In fact, one peculiar fact about garlic should be noted. Almost always it is the food of the poor people. Garlic was even used by the Babylonians about 3000 B.C.! All believed in the healing powers of garlic.

Used in
Olympics

The Greeks loved garlic. In fact the famous Greek philosopher Aristotle (384 B.C.) said of garlic:

> It is a cure for hydrophobia
> and as tonic,
> is a hot, laxative . . .

Hippocrates (460 B.C.) praised garlic as a medicine that promotes perspiration and both as a laxative and diuretic (medicine to aid in the secretion of urine).

Garlic was used in the Olympic Games by the athletes to increase their stamina.

The respected Roman physician, Galen (A.D. 131-200) spoke highly of garlic. Modern medicine considers Galen the father of medicine, incidentally. Galen believed that garlic helped to eradicate toxins from the bloodstream.

11

A RETURN TO NATURE'S REMEDIES

TIME FOR A CHANGE?

**The
Dark Age
Of Medicine**

It is only that as we became more "knowledgeable" that we substituted antibiotics.

Harry G. Bieler, M.D., in his book, <u>Food Is Your Best Medicine</u>, says:

> Today we are in the ... Antibiotic Age. Unhappily, too, this is the Dark Age of Medicine—an age in which many of my colleagues, when confronted with a patient, consult a volume which rivals the Manhattan telephone directory in size. This book contains the names of thousands upon thousands of drugs used to alleviate the distressing symptoms of a host of diseased states of the body. The doctor then decides which pink or purple or baby-blue pill to prescribe for the patient.[1]

As we near the close of the Twentieth Century, perhaps more doctors will see the value of old-fashioned remedies like garlic.

---
[1]Henry G. Bieler, M.D., <u>Food is Your Best Medicine</u> (New York: Random House), 1965, p. 13.

A Preservative

The Chinese used garlic to preserve fresh meat. In fact it has been found to have an antimicrobial effect on meat.

Cortez, conqueror of Mexico, discovered that the natives "*esteem garlic above all the roots of Europe.*"

For centuries the people of Bulgaria have made garlic a part of their daily diet! They chew garlic just as some people would chew tobacco. And Bulgarians are noted for their long life! Many of them still work a full day at 100 years of age. Could this remarkable herb, garlic, play an important part in the longevity of this very robust race of people?

A SOURCE FOR ENERGY

Provides Stamina and Strength

Garlic is still a mainstay in the Middle East. This tradition goes back to Egyptian days when Pharoah made sure the Israelites had plenty of garlic to eat. In the building of the pyramids, garlic was one of the main vegetables supplied in large quantities to the workers. In fact one of the first sit-down strikes to occur in history occurred during the building of the pyramid Cheops. They stopped working because their daily supply of garlic had been withheld! They knew they needed this herb for stamina, strength and endurance. If 5000 years ago common laborers knew the value of garlic, how much more enlightened should we be to its attributes now in the 20th Century!

Amazing Feats

Even today building and engineering experts are baffled as to how human energy was able to construct these colossal pyramids. Maybe if we ate garlic every day, we, too, could perform wonders!

Bibliography
Recommended Reading

Atkins, Robert C., M.D., *Dr. Atkins' Nutrition Breakthrough*, William Morrow and Company, Inc., New York, 1981.

Binding, G.J., *About Garlic*, Thorsons Publishers Limited, Wellingborough, Northamptonshire, England, 1970.

Bricklin, Mark, *The Practical Encyclopedia of Natural Healing*, Rodale Press, Emmaus, Pennsylvania, 1976.

Cooley, Donald G., *After-40 Health & Medical Guide*, Better Homes and Gardens Books, Des Moines, Iowa, 1980.

Harris, Lloyd J., *The Book of Garlic*, Holt, Rinehart and Winston, New York, 1975.

Hartshorn, Jeanette Charles, RN, BA, CCRN, *Hypertensive Crisis*, Nursing 80, Intermed Communications, Inc., Horsham, Penna., July, 1980.

Kirschmann, John D., *Nutrition Almanac*, McGraw-Hill Book Company, New York, 1975.

Miller, Sigmund S., *Symptoms*, Avon Books, New York, 1976.

Nourse, Alan E., M.D., *Ladies' Home Journal Family Medical Guide*, Harper & Row, New York, 1973.

Nurse's Guide To Drugs, Intermed Communications, Inc., Springhouse, Pennsylvania, 1981.

Rosenberg, Dr. Harold, *The Book of Vitamin Therapy*, Berkley Windhover Books, New York, 1974.

Whittlesey, Marietta, *Killer Salt*, Bolder Books, New York, 1977.

12

THE SECRET OF GARLIC

LEARNING FROM THE RUSSIANS

As Valuable As Money

To the Siberians garlic was as valuable as money. They paid their taxes in garlic; 5 bulbs for a child, 10 bulbs for a woman and 15 bulbs for a man. That gives me an idea. I think I'll pay my income tax in garlic bulbs. The nation may be healthier for it!

Russian Penicillin

The Chinese and the Russians do not shy away from old-fashioned remedies for illness. In fact, Soviet scientists use what is termed "Russian Penicillin." It is a distillation of garlic (Allicin) which kills only unhealthy bacteria and leaves the natural healthy bacteria alone, reports Lloyd J. Harris, in his excellent book, The Book of Garlic.

Doctors used garlic extensively during the 18th and 19th centuries. However, since World War 2, we have changed over from natural healing herbal remedies to drugs. Prior to World War 2, patients were not bombarded with an avalanche of drugs. Herbal medicines were respected. They had no side effects and patients did not become addicts. They received treatment as God provided it, right from the earth!

**A
Common
Remedy**

It may be hard for some to realize that every plant is a miracle. And many doctors are now coming to realize garlic's medicinal power. Garlic is a strong antiseptic, a germicidal agent and has disease-preventative qualities. For centuries, garlic has been a common remedy for colds in many European countries.

Studies in the University of Geneva have indicated that blood pressure was effectively lowered in many patients who had high blood pressure and included garlic in their diet. Garlic appears to open blood vessels, thus reducing the blood pressure. In these same studies patients noted that dizziness, angina and headaches often disappeared!

13

GARLIC . . . THE FOUNTAIN OF YOUTH?

**Garlic's
Secret
Ingredient**

Garlic is an antiseptic. It is credited with saving thousands of lives in World War 1.

While garlic is rich in vitamins and minerals, its secret powers lie in only 2% content of the product—that which makes it smell. It is called allyd disulphate. This potent, essential, natural oil is the power behind the throne! It is nature's penicillin!

**For
Failing
Memory**

What medicinal properties are attributed to garlic! Mrs. Eleanor Roosevelt, at a late age, was asked what was the secret of her remarkable memory.

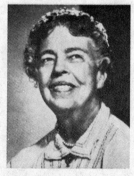

She replied: "Garlic cloves!"

She had read that garlic was an old, folk remedy for failing memory. So she faithfully consumed three honey-covered cloves every morning.

OTHER BLESSINGS

For Asthma

Farmers in England use garlic as a remedy for asthma. Others rub pimples and other skin irritations with garlic several times a day. They claim this makes the skin problem disappear without leaving any scars! Garlic is considered a sedative for the stomach. Most people prefer to take garlic in capsule form because of its strong flavor.

I can still picture my mother using garlic in making that famous Lebanese salad called Tabbouleh (pronounced tah-boo-lee).[1] We lived on a little farm in Schultzville, Pennsylvania near Clarks Summit and Scranton. It was the depression days of the early 1930's. Garlic to us was gold . . . more precious than gold! The preparation of this salad was almost a ritual.

My mother would get a large garlic bulb, peel the cloves, then slice the cloves real thin. These slices would be put into a large cup with just a covering of pure olive oil. For several minutes she would painstakingly crush the slices of garlic until the aroma had penetrated the olive oil.

---

[1]The recipe for Tabbouleh can be found in **HOW TO EAT YOUR WAY BACK TO VIBRANT HEALTH** by Salem Kirban. Send $6 (includes postage) to: Salem Kirban, Inc., Kent Road, Huntingdon Valley, Pennsylvania 19006.

When this was done, she would add more olive oil, filling the cup. The essence of garlic-oil would then be stirred to permeate the entire contents. The ritual was completed. Prior to this she had prepared all the other ingredients for the Tabbouleh salad.

Liquid Gold

Carefully she poured this liquid gold over the salad. And then the secret! She left the salad "rest" for one day in our ice box. Overnight the garlic was celebrating a marriage as it wedded itself to the parsley, the scallions, the mint, the bulgur wheat and the tomatoes. What a wedding!

The next day . . . what a feast! It was a food too good for the selective palates of Presidents and Kings and Queens. It was a food for we peasants, who didn't have two dimes to rub together, for we knew the secret of God's garlic. Yes, if I had to choose between gold and garlic, I would choose GARLIC . . . for it is nature's GOLD!

GARLIC SOUP
8 Servings

Who ever heard of garlic soup? One might think this would have a very strong garlic flavor . . . but it is surprisingly mild. It is a refreshing winter soup and so beneficial for you. And garlic is so cheap!

With a joy and zest for living, go down to your supermarket and quickly grab:

2 large heads fresh garlic

Tenderly separate the heads of garlic into cloves. Place the cloves in a cup and while they are not looking, pour boiling water all over them! Then undress them by slipping off their skins. Now drop them in a kettle with:

- **2 quarts water**
- **2 tablespoons sea salt**
- **¼ teaspoon cayenne pepper**
- **2 whole cloves**
- **¼ teaspoon sage**
- **¼ teaspoon thyme**
- **5 sprigs parsley**
- **2 tablespoons oil**

Bring to a boil and then let simmer for 30 minutes.

Awaken the chicken and take from her:

- **3 eggs**
- **¼ cup melted butter**

Beat these together vigorously so they get fully acquainted and become fast friends. Meanwhile, back at the ranch, take that simmering pot with all the water in it and strain the soup mixture. To the strained liquid, slowly add the egg mixture beating the liquid with vigor as you add. Reheat but do not boil. Your soup is now ready to partake.

If you want to live dangerously, don't bother straining the soup. Sip up the dregs and all!

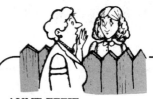

AUNT EFFIE . . .
Poor Alphonso has arteriosclerosis!

That's just a big name for hardening of the arteries! Several things happen and it just doesn't occur overnight. Your blood vessels are like the new pipes you installed in your house. You start running some adulterated water through and over the years lime deposits build up and the inside diameter of the pipe narrows. Same with Alphonso's blood vessels. Wrong eating habits, slowly over the years, have made his arteries become thick with gunk. The passage way for the blood becomes narrower, the walls of the blood vessels lose their elasticity. Soon he becomes forgetful. Blood pressure increases. He gets cramps in his legs and notices circulation problems.

Atherosclerosis is a form of arteriosclerosis and both are no bonanza! They cause most of the heart attacks and strokes. So Alphonso better "fasta from the pasta." Did you know he wears a girdle? A girdle is a device to keep an unfortunate situation from spreading!

Granny Osgood has a good remedy for high blood pressure and artery problems. She drinks 4 ounces of carrot juice mixed with 3 ounces of pineapple juice. She drinks this and eats three honey-covered garlic cloves every morning. Alphonso may want to substitute garlic perles he can buy at the health food store.

14

GARLIC AND YOUR BLOOD PRESSURE

GARLIC TESTS PROMISING

**Lowered
Blood
Pressure**

Various medical sources in France and Germany discovered that garlic lowered blood pressure in some 40% of their cases. Garlic opened up blood vessels, thus reducing pressure. It stopped angina pains and dizziness.

In 1915, during World War 1, E. E. Marcovici, an army doctor on the Eastern front, carried out many experiments with garlic. He continued prescribing garlic for 25 years thereafter successfully and reported his findings in the January, 1941 *Medical Record.*[1]

Marcovici found garlic effective against High Blood Pressure. Previous garlic studies reported that garlic had a vasodilatory effect on blood vessels ... that is, it widens them. Marcovici claimed that garlic's power was its ability to control and purify intestinal putrefaction. Marcovici worked with the elderly who had High Blood Pressure and found that most of them suffered from chronic constipation, appendicitis and retention of

[1]E. E. Marcovici, Garlic Therapy For Digestive Disorders, *(Medical Record)*, 153:63-65, January, 1941

fecal waste in the bowels. Because of this, the toxins were absorbed into the blood stream ... causing symptoms of headache, dizziness, fatigue and capillary spasms.

Promotes Bowel Regularity

By concentrating on getting the bowels moving with regularity, garlic became a valuable treatment to High Blood Pressure.[1]

ENCOURAGING REPORTS

For A Healthier Bowel

In 1941, Emil Weiss in Chicago, reported that garlic treatments caused healthful bacteria in the intestine to increase while symptoms of headache and diarrhea vanished.[2]

Frederic Damsau also worked with garlic to lower blood pressure. Damsau reaffirmed the link between garlic's ability to control putrefaction (build up of bowel wastes) and the lowering of blood pressure.[3]

Two cardiologists, Drs. Bordi and Bansal, of the Department of Medicine, R.N.T.

[1]Lloyd J. Harris, The Book of Garlic (New York: Holt, Rinehart and Winston), 1975, p. 106.

[2]Emil Weiss, A Clinical Study of the Effects of Desiccated Garlic in Intestinal Flora, (Medical Record) 153:404-8, June, 1941.

[3]Frederic Damsau, The Use of Garlic Concentrate in Vascular Hypertension, (Medical Record) 153:249-51, April, 1941.

Medical College, Udaipur, India found garlic useful in lowering blood cholesterol and fibrinogen levels to a safe level. Fibrinogen is a protein present in blood plasma which causes blood to clot.

Combats Drug Side Effects

The two doctors, after their tests, concluded:

> *Clinically, garlic could avoid most of these drawbacks* [the drawbacks of side effects of drugs] *and could be recommended for long-term use without danger of toxicity.*[1]

Liquid Garlic

Garlic is available in tablet and capsule form. While many object to the smell and taste of garlic, Japanese have discovered a way to eliminate the odor. This liquid garlic comes in perles or capsules. Some nutritionists recommend taking 5 or 6 capsules a day with meals.[2]

---

[1] *The Lancet*, December 29, 1973, pp. 1491-2.

[2] Many nutritionists believe that *"Death starts in the colon."* They suggest that constipation and poor bowel habits over the years causes both a build-up and back-up of toxins that first show their sign in high blood pressure and eventually in a serious illness. **For further information, you may wish a copy of BOWEL PROBLEMS by Salem Kirban.** Send $5 (plus $1 for postage) to: Salem Kirban, Inc., Kent Road, Huntingdon Valley, Pennsylvania 19006.

The heart: a muscular pump

Inside the heart

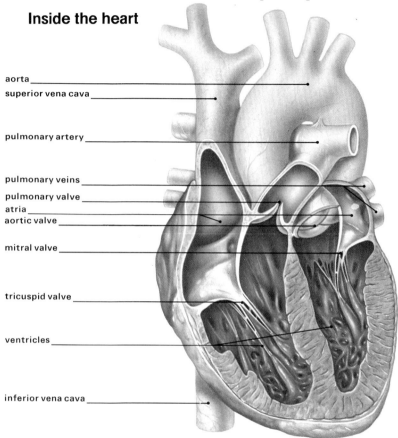

aorta

superior vena cava

pulmonary artery

pulmonary veins

pulmonary valve

atria

aortic valve

mitral valve

tricuspid valve

ventricles

inferior vena cava

The heart is a muscular pumping organ which beats nonstop to circulate blood around the body. It functions as **two** halves, each consisting of a holding chamber, or atrium, and a pumping center, or ventricle.

After circulating around the body, blood, now deoxygenated, returns to the right atrium through large veins, the superior vena cava and the inferior vena cava. When the atrium is full, blood is forced through the tricuspid valve into the right ventricle. It is then pumped to the lungs through the pulmonary valve into the pulmonary artery.

The oxygenated blood returns via the pulmonary veins to the left atrium. After flowing through the mitral valve it is pumped out of the left ventricle into the aorta to return to the general circulation.

Mitchell Beazley Publishers, Ltd., England
Atlas of the Body and Mind, Copyright: Mitchell Beazley Publishers, Ltd.
1976. Published in U.S.A. by Rand McNally & Company.

The stomach

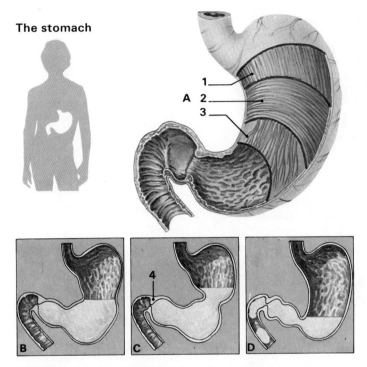

The stomach acts as a reservoir for food and has a capacity of two and a half pints. Within the stomach, solid food material is churned and kneaded for about three hours until it becomes a semiliquid mass known as chyme. The chyme is then forced into the small intestine, where the process of digestion is completed. The wall of the stomach (**A**) has three muscular layers, an outer longitudinal layer (**1**), a middle circular layer (**2**) and an inner oblique layer (**3**) As the stomach fills with food, wavelike contractions of the wall begin (**B**), and as these waves move along the stomach wall (**C**) some of the food is passed through the relaxed muscle valve at the base (**4**) and into the duodenum (**D**), the first part of the small intestine, where it is further digested before being absorbed into the body.

Mitchell Beazley Publishers, Ltd., England Atlas of the Body and Mind, Copyright © Mitchell Beazley Publishers, Ltd. 1976. Published in U.S.A. by Rand McNally & Company.

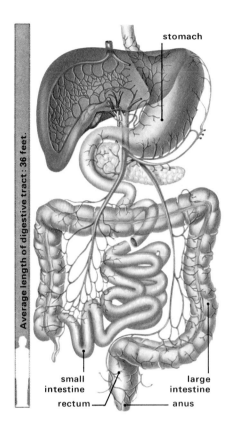

Average length of digestive tract: 36 feet.

stomach

small
intestine

large
intestine

rectum

anus

The digestive system

From the mouth, food passes
down the throat into the
stomach, where a churning
action mixes it into a
semiliquid mass.

It is then forced into the
small intestine, where the
major part of digestion and
absorption occurs.

Undigested material passes
into the large intestine, where
most of the remaining water is
absorbed by the bloodstream.

Solid waste collects in the
rectum and is expelled
through the anus.

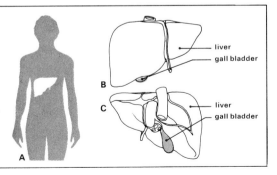

The liver and gall bladder are
positioned close to each other high up in
the abdomen (**A**). In the front view (**B**),
the gall bladder cannot be clearly seen as
it lies tucked underneath the liver. In the
back view of the liver (**C**), however, the
pear-shaped gall bladder is clearly
visible. The liver produces bile juice,
which passes down the hepatic duct to
be stored in the gall bladder. Periodically,
bile is released into the duodenum,
where it aids the digestion of fats and
neutralizes the acidity of chyme—food
partly digested in the stomach.

liver

gall bladder

B

C

liver

gall bladder

A

The pacemaker of the heart, a tiny area of specialized nervous tissue in the right atrium, sets the heart beating about seventy times a minute. Without it the heart would beat only forty times per minute, which is too slow for the body's needs. The pacemaker, or sinuatrial node (**1**), regularly sends out nerve impulses which spread through the two atria, causing them to contract. From the atrioventricular node (**2**) the contraction spreads down special conducting tissue, the bundle of His (**3**), causing the ventricles to contract and pump blood out of the heart.

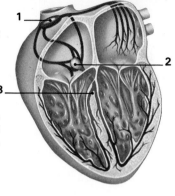

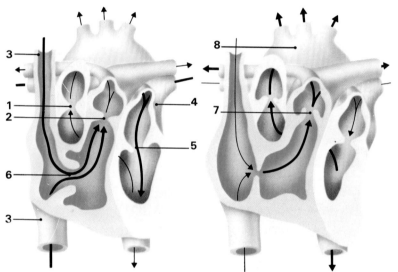

With each heartbeat there are <u>two</u> phases in the passage of oxygenated blood (<u>red</u>) and deoxygenated blood (<u>blue</u>) through the heart.

In the phase of relaxation, or diastole (left), the heart fills with blood. As the ventricles relax, valves in the aorta (**1**) and in the pulmonary artery (**2**) close with a dup sound and blood pours into the two atria from the venae cavae (**3**) and the pulmonary veins (**4**). The mitral (**5**) and tricuspid (**6**) valves between the atria and ventricles open, allowing blood into the ventricles. The heart then stops filling with blood.

In the phase of contraction, or systole (right), the heart empties and a lub sound is made by the closing of the mitral and tricuspid valves. This prevents a backflow of blood into the atria as it is pumped from the ventricles into the pulmonary artery (**7**) and aorta (**8**).

Each heartbeat lasts for up to eight-tenths of a second, with systole lasting for four-tenths of a second and diastole occupying the remaining time.

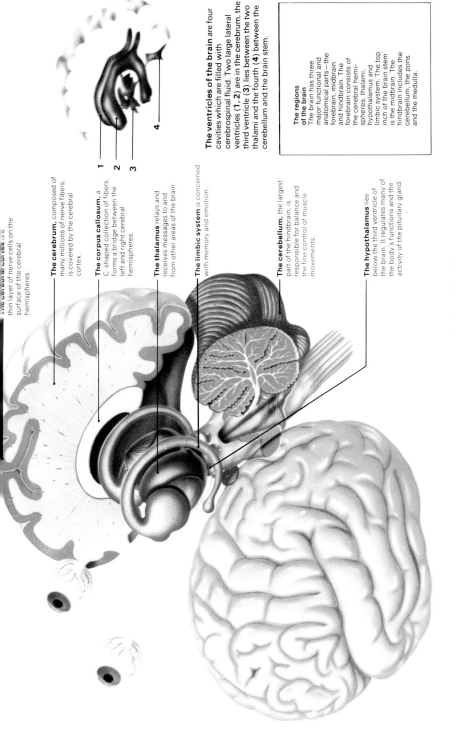

The cerebral cortex is a thin layer of nerve cells on the surface of the cerebral hemispheres.

The cerebrum, composed of many millions of nerve fibers, is covered by the cerebral cortex.

The corpus callosum, a C-shaped collection of fibers, forms a bridge between the left and right cerebral hemispheres.

The thalamus relays and receives messages to and from other areas of the brain.

The limbic system is concerned with memory and emotion.

The cerebellum, the largest part of the hindbrain, is responsible for balance and the fine control of muscle movements.

The hypothalamus lies below the third ventricle of the brain. It regulates many of the body's functions and the activity of the pituitary gland.

The ventricles of the brain are four cavities which are filled with cerebrospinal fluid. Two large lateral ventricles (1, 2) are in the cerebrum, the third ventricle (3) lies between the two thalami and the fourth (4) between the cerebellum and the brain stem.

The regions of the brain
The brain has three major functional and anatomical parts—the forebrain, midbrain and hindbrain. The forebrain consists of the cerebral hemispheres, thalami, hypothalamus and limbic system. The top inch of the brain stem is the midbrain. The hindbrain includes the cerebellum, the pons and the medulla.

KIDNEYS: filtration units

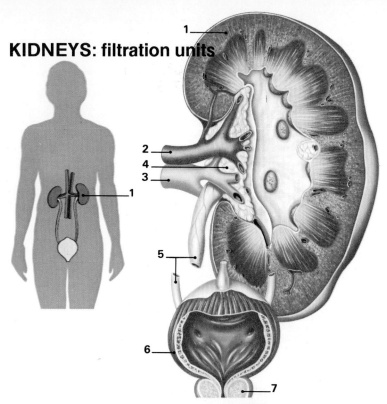

The urinary system is concerned with the formation and elimination of urine. In an adult, more than 2,500 pints of blood pass through the kidneys (**1**) each day.

Blood enters via the renal arteries (**2**) and is filtered to remove most of the waste products of metabolism. Seven pints of filtrate are produced every hour. Purified blood returns to the body circulation via the renal veins (**3**). The filtering process is carried out by more than two million tiny kidney units, or nephrons, which produce a highly concentrated solution of chemicals known as urine, which is harmful to the body if allowed to remain. Urine flows from the nephrons, first into the funnel-shaped renal pelvis (**4**) and then into the ureter (**5**).

Waves of muscular contraction passing down the ureters push the urine into the bladder (**6**). With continuous filling, the bladder, a muscular bag, expands until it holds about one pint of fluid. A circular band of muscle around the neck of the bladder, the sphincter (**7**), controls the release of urine from the body.

Mitchell Beazley Publishers, Ltd., England Atlas of the Body and Mind, Copyright © Mitchell Beazley Publishers, Ltd. 1976. Published in U.S.A. by Rand McNally & Company.

Barriers To Infection

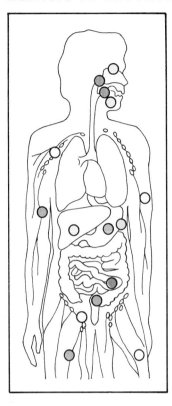

Lachrymal glands, above the outer corner of each eye, secrete tears, which wash dust and dirt from the eyes. They contain chemicals that kill bacteria.

Tonsils and adenoids are composed of lymphoid tissue. Located at the entrances to the throat, they act as barriers to bacteria and viruses.

Salivary glands are found in the cheeks and under the tongue. The saliva they secrete contains substances which help to resist infection.

Lymph nodes are small glands which produce white blood cells. Some of these cells produce antibodies and others ingest bacteria.

The lymphatic system carries tissue fluid, or lymph, around the body. Lymph contains white cells and carries bacteria to the lymph nodes, where they are trapped and destroyed.

The liver produces some of the factors which make blood clot and so initiate wound repair.

The stomach produces hydrochloric acid, which sterilizes ingested food and kills bacteria.

The spleen, composed of lymphoid tissue, produces white blood cells and removes unwanted debris from the blood.

The small intestine is usually sterile, for bacteria have previously been killed by gastric acid and broken down by digestive enzymes.

The large intestine contains harmless bacteria which effectively exclude harmful bacteria from colonizing.

The skin is the body's main protection against disease. Invasion of organisms through the skin only occurs when it is damaged.

The three main routes of entry to the body for agents of disease are (**1**) through wounds, (**2**) by inhalation and (**3**) by ingestion. The skin is the first line of defense. The air we breathe is full of potentially harmful organisms but the respiratory system is designed to trap and remove any invaders. The tonsils and adenoids form a protective ring of tissue around the entrance to the throat. White blood cells in the blood and lymphatic system also fight infection.

The Regulation of Metabolism

The pituitary gland controls the metabolism of fats, carbohydrates and proteins by releasing growth hormone and by controlling hormone output of the thyroid gland.

The Thyroid gland controls the metabolic rate of the body. It manufactures the hormones thyroxine, which affects the rate of chemical reactions in the cells.

The liver controls the supply of nutrients to the cells. In particular it sieves carbohydrates from the blood and regulates the amount of glucose in the circulation.

The pancreas secretes the hormones insulin and glucagon, which affect carbohydrate metabolism and, to a lesser extent, fat and protein metabolism.

The overall metabolism of the body is governed and constantly monitored by various organs of the body which are anatomically separate, but which function as a complete unit.

Metabolism involves chemical changes which convert food we eat into the components of the body, or burn food to provide energy.

Within each body cell digested carbohydrate, fat and protein are finally reduced to a relatively simple substance called acetyl coenzyme A.

During his lifetime the average man eats about fifty tons of food and yet maintains a weight of about 160 pounds. Even the most obese person retains in his body only a minute fraction of what he eats. Most of the food we absorb into our bodies through the process of digestion must sooner or later pass out again.

Few nutrients leave the body unchanged. Most are modified or interconverted in one of the multitude of chemical pathways that are described as metabolism. The breakdown of nutrients is the prerequisite of life, since the energy required to keep the body going comes from this breakdown.

In some ways the body is exactly like a flame—fuel (food) is burned, using oxygen from the air, releasing energy as heat or for work. Indeed, the fuels of food can be burned in an ordinary fire. In all the body, however, they are burned slowly and step by step, so that the energy of the fire of life is released a little at a time in a way that is the most useful.

This stepwise regulation of metabolism is achieved by the thousands of different kinds of giant molecules of protein, called enzymes, which are found in all the cells of the body. It is enzymes that make body chemistry work at all, since the fire of life not only burns slowly but also burns in the internal environment of the body, which is three-quarters water.

15

B VITAMINS BENEFICIAL

Vitamin B₁

Vitamin B_1 *(thiamine)*, Choline and Folic Acid have been found to be beneficial for those suffering from heart disease.

Vitamin B₃

The Mayo Clinic has given Vitamin B_3 (Niacin) to those with high cholesterol blood levels. Both the Canadian Medical Association Journal and British Medical Journal in 1957, 1958 included articles by physicians showing they had established that Niacin was a valuable anti-cholesterol agent. A new version of Niacin (Niacinamide) does not cause flushing of the skin as Niacin does.

B-vitamins are water soluble and non-toxic. The B-complex vitamins, for the most part, are dependent upon one another for their interrelation. Therefore it is better to take them all together in one supplement.

Vitamin B₆

Dr. Kilmer McCully, professor of pathology at Harvard Medical School, on the basis of extensive laboratory studies, is convinced that the underlying cause of arteriosclerosis is caused by a series of events initiated by a deficiency of pyridoxine, which is Vitamin B_6. Dr. McCully believes that both Vitamin B_6 and the amino acid methionine are essential elements in preventing arteriosclerosis. He also believes that B_6 may partially reverse damage already done.

While B_6 is found in many foods, it is sensitive to heat. Thus it is often destroyed by the cook, the canner and the food processor. Bananas and carrots have the highest desired ratios of B_6 with the amino acid methionine. The elderly are often highly deficient in these nutrients thus encouraging heart disease.

Many researchers feel that 25-50 milligrams of B_6 provide the best safeguard against heart disease, so long as the vitamin is taken in conjunction with other B-complex vitamins to keep them in balance.

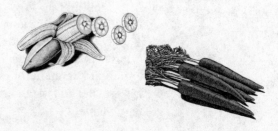

16

VITAMIN E AND BLOOD PRESSURE

VITAMIN E

**Sprouts
Are
Best
Source**

Much has been written about Vitamin E. It has been hailed as the *Youth Vitamin* as the greatest concentration of Vitamin E is found in fresh, young seed sprouts. Vitamin E is essential for more youthful strength, vitality, good health and reproductive ability.

Vitamin E is a natural anti-thrombin. Thrombin is the enzyme in the blood that causes blood clots. Vitamin E prevents internal blood clots.

**Aids
Heart**

Vitamin E is a natural anti-oxidant. It provides what is called an oxygen sparing action. Vitamin E is able to decrease the oxygen requirement of the heart muscle by as much as 43%. This oxygen *"rationing"* by Vitamin E reduces fatigue and helps your heart from being overworked.

Vitamin E aids in prevention of harmful and excessive scar tissue. It is also a dilator of blood vessels opening them up to provide new pathways for damaged circulation.

**Many Nutritionists believe
SPROUTS PROVIDE YOUR
HIGHEST VITAMIN CONTENT
Naturally!**

Sprouts are actually described as *"perfect"* because all the life-giving proteins, carbohydrates, oils, vitamins and minerals necessary to support our life system are stored within the seed itself.

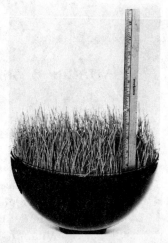

When seeds begin to sprout, their vitamin content accelerates at a remarkable rate. The first shoots of soybeans (per 100 grams of seed) contain about 100 milligrams of vitamin C, but after 72 hours the content soars to approximately 700 milligrams, an increase of almost 700 percent! **This means that soybean sprouts contain almost 20 times the amount of vitamin C that is provided in a glass of orange juice!** Similar comparisons can be made for most of the vitamins, including Vitamin A, the B vitamins and E.

Sprouts satisfy one's need for protein without consuming high calories. One ounce of meat, both lean and fat, contains approximately 80 calories . . . whereas one ounce of beansprouts has only about 10 calories and . . . contains no cholesterol!

There are some health clinics that specialize in "wheat grass therapy" in their approach to cancer patients. Many believe that sprouts are part of the answer to stopping the ravages of cancer and starting the healing process.

Sprouted seeds, the very beginning of new life, are one of the highest forms of nutrition known. They are free of chemical additives. You can grow them in your kitchen in just 12 inches of space! And you can have a harvest of nutritious home grown sprouts every 3 to 4 days.

There's a double bonus, too. Not only do you benefit by the nutritious value of sprouts, but you also save on your food bill.

CHECK WITH DOCTOR

**A Word
Of
Caution**

A doctor should determine the amount of Vitamin E for each heart patient. **Rheumatic fever patients should not take Vitamin E without their doctor's approval.**

As a health maintenance vitamin, 800 to 1600 Units (I.U.) daily is recommended by many nutritionists. Some doctors routinely prescribe 100 I.U.s of Vitamin E three times a day to hospital patients undergoing surgery or who are prone to blood clots.[1]

Nutritionists recommend that the Vitamin E you take is natural and not synthetic. Natural E's include d-Alpha Tocopherol and "*Mixed tocopherols*"—with d-Alpha being most popular.

**Under
Medical
Supervision**

Dr. Wilfrid Shute has said that Vitamin E therapy often helps patients with high blood pressure, but he always makes certain that the condition has stabilized before giving supplements. Patients with uncontrolled blood pressure may have an adverse reaction. In an informal survey taken by Prevention magazine, a surprising number of people had reduced their blood pressure significantly after taking Vitamin E over an extended period of

[1]Alton Ochsner, M.D., New England Journal of Medicine, July 23, 1964.

**Please
Read
Carefully!**

time, with the typical dose falling into the range of about 400 to 800 I.U. a day.[1]

Those with rheumatic heart conditions should **not** take supplementary Vitamin E except under medical supervision. High Blood Pressure cases should, upon approval of your physician, begin with small doses (100 I.U.) and have their blood pressure carefully monitored as the dosage increases. (Since Vitamin E improves the efficiency of the heart, it can drive the blood pressure up in hypertensive patients, though it does not have this effect on others.) Rheumatic heart fever sufferers have an imbalance between the two sides of the heart. Large Vitamin E doses can increase the imbalance, worsening the patient's condition. The alpha-tocopherol fraction of the tocopherol compounds has the most Vitamin E activity. For this vitamin, 1 I.U. (International Unit) is the same as 1 milligram.[2]

---

[1]Mark Bricklin, Natural Healing, (Emmaus, Pennsylvania: Rodale Press), 1978, p. 60.

[2]Dr. Harold Rosenberg, The Book of Vitamin Therapy, (New York: Berkley Windhover Books), 1974, p. 98, 99.

17

MINERALS AND YOUR BLOOD PRESSURE

ZINC

Cadmium Buildup Dangerous

People who eat refined foods such as white flour, rice and white sugar are taking into their bodies a toxic range of Cadmium. Cadmium is a toxic trace mineral that has many structural similarities to zinc. Therefore, its toxic effects are kept under control in the body by the presence of zinc. Refining processes, unfortunately, disturb the important cadmium-zinc balance.

For example, whole wheat has a zinc to cadmium ratio of over 100 to one. But after that whole wheat has been "enriched," the ratio drops to about 17 to one. The same is true for rice and probably other grains.

In addition, cigarette smoke and automobile exhaust emit cadmium. Runoff water from mines, as well as waste water from industry, puts cadmium into the water and from there to our food supply.

Zinc is found in the following foods:

Sunflower seeds
Seafood
Mushrooms
Brewer's yeast
Soybeans

Zinc Supplements

Nutritionists recommend that zinc supplements be taken with calcium or bone meal for better absorption. A zinc supplement of 15-30 milligrams a day are recommended by some.[1] Zinc gluconate is more readily absorbed than zinc sulfate.

Coffee and commercial teas contain high levels of cadmium. Softening water also seems to increase the amount of cadmium entering the body. Hair samples taken from residents of a soft water area were found to contain an average of 6.6 parts per million of cadmium. The normal range is between .1 and 1.6 ppm.

When a deficit of Zinc occurs in the diet, the body may make it up by storing Cadmium instead.[2]

Dr. Henry A. Shroeder, a trace mineral researcher, has developed a theory about cadmium being a major causative factor in High Blood Pressure and related heart ailments. He found that regular high doses of cadmium caused increased tension. The urine of hypertensive patients contains up to 40% more cadmium than does the urine of persons with normal blood pressure.[3]

---

[1]Dr. Harold Rosenberg, The Book of Vitamin Therapy, (New York: Berkley Windhover Books), 1974, p. 172.

[2]John D. Kirschmann, Nutrition Almanac, (New York: McGraw-Hill Book Company), 1975, p. 62.

[3]Complete Book of Minerals for Health, (Emmaus, Pennsylvania: Rodale Press), pp. 413, 277.

1
The MINERAL Approach To Illness
An Interview with Paul Eck

Dr. Paul Eck has a degree in the field of naprapathy. Naprapathy is a system of therapy which attributes all disease to disorders of the nervous system, ligaments and connective tissue.

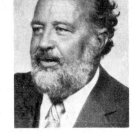

He is director of Analytical Research Laboratories in Phoenix, Arizona which specializes in interpreting hair tests. Paul Eck prepares vitamin and mineral programs for many medical doctors and other health practitioners.

Dr. Eck has very definite views on how to correct basic illnesses. They differ quite dramatically from the standard medical approach to disease. In fact, they differ also from many of the usual nutritional approaches to disease, as well!

Dr. Eck believes that much of what is going on today in the field of nutrition is guesswork. Too many people are spending anywhere from $5000 to $15,000 to correct health deficiences and are no better off physically. The problem, as Eck sees it, is that it is not the products they are taking that are wrong . . . but that the necessary knowledge and application to utilize these various nutrients is missing!

In an interview with Sam and Loren Biser of The Healthview Newsletter, Eck commented:

> It's not the amount of vitamins that you take nor is it the amount of minerals you are taking or anything else . . . the products or the money that you are spending . . . I think a lot of this is pure waste because if it is not being applied in a scientific way there's no way that it's ever going to work![1]

---

[1] Paul Eck, Your Minerals and Your Health (To secure this one hour cassette, send $10 direct to Healthview Newsletter, Box 6670, Charlottesville, Virginia 22906)

Other cassettes by Dr. Paul Eck on various metabolic dysfunctions and philosophy of health are available from Analytical Research Laboratories, Inc., 2338 West Royal Palm Road, Suite F, Phoenix, Arizona 85021.

The MINERAL Approach To Illness
An Interview with Paul Eck

Paul Eck is a firm believer in using hair analysis tests.

A hair analysis test is the only method developed that has any validity at all as far as measuring what actually is occurring in the tissues of the body.

It has the benefit of being able to give you a metabolic pattern of every metabolic activity that is occurring in your body over a period of time.[1]

Dr. Eck believes that blood tests, in this context, are frequently invalid because they give you an up-to-the-minute readout. It is not a true reflection of what is happening in the tissues over a period of time. A person taking a high amount of Vitamin C could be releasing from his system large amounts of cholesterol. If a blood test were taken at that time it would show a high cholesterol level. However, what the physician does not realize is that it is not a build-up of cholesterol but, quite the opposite, a beneficial flushing of cholesterol out of the body.

Too many people, Dr. Eck suggests, take maganese when they have a manganese deficiency . . . they take iron when they have an iron deficiency, etc. **This is wrong.** To give iron to raise iron is to lower iron!

Dr. Louis Kervan, in his book, Biological Transmutations makes the following observations:

For IRON deficiency . . . give Manganese.
For MANGANESE deficiency . . . give Copper.
For MAGNESIUM deficiency . . . give Zinc.
For ZINC deficiency . . . give Magnesium.

High Blood Pressure

As with numerous chronic metabolic dysfunctions . . . hypertension has many cuases with as many mineral indicators. Although each of these indicators are of great significance, the sodium/potassium ratio is particularly significant.

The optimal ratio is **2.5** parts of sodium to **one** part of potassium. When the sodium/potassium ratio is chronically greater than **10/1,** there exists a water retention in the tissues, this creates stress, kidney overload, and many other conditions which contribute to, and are associated with hypertension.

[1]Ibid.

3
The MINERAL Approach To Illness
An Interview with Paul Eck

When you go on a correct vitamin/ mineral supplementation, the excess minerals and toxic minerals (such as cadmium, lead, aluminum) will start to unload and flush out of your system. This unloading will cause headaches and numerous other symptoms which will vary with the toxic metal or combination of toxic metals being eliminated, and in some cases make you feel worse. This is a natural occurrence as your body gets rid of these unwanted elements to get you on the road to full recovery.

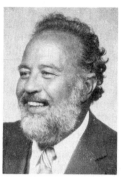

Dr. Eck believes that mineral imbalances should be corrected mainly by using <u>small</u> potency vitamins and minerals. He says it just takes a very small amount of a mineral to initiate a major physiological process in the body. Any amount over that, he states, will cause exactly the opposite reaction.

Paul Eck believes that mineral therapy is also indirectly hormone therapy. Through the results found in hair analysis he has been able to see people go off hormone therapy, estrogen, even off of thyroxin. He has used manganese and copper to improve their thyroid function where indicated.

Paul Eck is very familiar with Diabetes. His grandmother, his mother was diabetic. He and his brother were pre-diabetic. Dr. Eck states he can determine from a hair analysis, years in advance, whether a person will become a diabetic.

Paul Eck says that 90% of the people who have diabetes have more than enough insulin circulating in their blood. When you have a low calcium to magnesium ratio (such as 3.3 to 1) you have an individual that has diabetes. And if the ratio is high, such as <u>10</u> parts calcium to <u>1</u> part magnesium . . . you are in the diabetic area.[1]

Eck states:

> *One problem in about 10% of the diabetics is the lack of calcium in the pancreas. This condition results in an inability of the Islets of Langerhans to secrete insulin . . .*

[1]The calcium to magnesium <u>ratio</u> normally is 6.7 to 1. This means for every 1 part of magnesium in your system, you should have 6.7 parts of calcium.

because when the calcium drops below a certain level you can't even initiate the secretion of the insulin that is manufactured and is being stored in pancreatic Islets of Langerhans tissue.

So what you have to do is, by one means or another, raise the calcium level back up to a close to normal ratio between the magnesium and then you automatically get a secretion of insulin.

This occurs in your insulin-deficiency diabetics ... which only accounts for about 10 or 12% of the cases.

Dr. Eck states that the rest of the problem in diabetes lies either in the transport of the insulin to the cell itself or, when it gets to the cell, there is a lack of a receptor at the cell site on the cell membrane. Those receptors are all minerals! Therefore, Dr. Eck concludes:

If the proper mineral is not available in the body for transport of the insulin to the cell ... it doesn't get there in the first place.

Secondly, even when it gets there, if some receptor is not present, and there are multiple receptors on the cell membrane ... then, of course, the insulin can't even enter the cell and do what it is supposed to do!

We have had such great reports especially in diabetes.

You know the old saying that says "Once you've been on insulin, you're going to stay on it the rest of your life ..."
that's the same statement they use for hypothyroidism. They say: "Once you're on thyroid, you're going to be on it forever. Make up your mind to it."

Some individuals have been able to have their insulin requirement reduced or completely eliminated within a few weeks. These, of course, are spectacular cases. There are also insulin-taking diabetics who require a year or two to bring about a complete correction. The individual must be extremely cooperative. Attempts to correct diabetes must be done under the supervision of a doctor.

Dr. Eck says that those taking oral hypoglycemic agents for diabetics are the easiest cases to correct. Correcting those with juvenile diabetes is much more difficult ... unless the individual faithfully stays on the health program.

If the ratio remains chronic . . . Dr. Eck believes there are $\underline{7}$ mineral clues as to whether a person is developing cancer. The more of these clues they have the more severe their condition is. Here are the clues:

*1. Calcium/Magnesium ratio of <u>less than</u> 2 parts of calcium to 1 part of magnesium . . . is a cancer indicator.

*2. Calcium/Magnesium ratio of <u>over</u> 14 parts of calcium to 1 part of magnesium . . . is a cancer indicator.

*3. Sodium/Potassium inversion. Normally sodium is $\underline{25}$ in ratio to your potassium, which is $\underline{10}$. This is a 2.5 to 1 sodium to potassium ratio. If the ratio inverts (goes <u>lower</u> than 1.5 to 1) this could be indicative of cancer, kidney disease, hypertension, infections, osteoarthritis, etc.!

*4. Zinc/copper ratio of <u>over</u> 16 parts of zinc to 1 part of copper . . . is a cancer indicator.

*5. Zinc/copper ratio of <u>less than</u> 4 parts of zinc to 1 part of copper . . . is a cancer indicator.

*6. <u>Copper</u> greater than 10 and less than 1.0 irregardless of ratios . . . is a cancer indicator.

*7. <u>Iron</u> greater than 10 and less than 1.0 . . . is a cancer indicator.

Paul Eck believes that there are important interrelationships between minerals and vitamins. An excess of one mineral can cause an imbalance in another mineral in your body. Such imbalances can lead to illness. Here are some examples:

1. MANGANESE

Manganese can lower <u>magnesium</u> levels in the body if your magnesium level is already low, the additional lowering by taking manganese can cause epileptic seizures and other neuro-muscular dysfunctions.

2. CALCIUM

Whenever you take large amounts of calcium, Eck states you will lose potassium. He says about 80% of the people in the United States suffer from a sluggish thyroid. This causes a high blood cholesterol, lack of incentive, fatigue. Eck says:

---

*These ratios figures are Paul Eck's testing figures. They are not standard ratio figures. What other testing laboratories for hair analysis may consider a normal ratio . . . Eck may consider not in the normal range.

Potassium is necessary for thyroxin, which is a hormone of the thyroid gland.

Therefore, if one takes calcium causing a lowering in potassium he will have a lowering of thryoid function.

Calcium will also drive magnesium out of the body causing a high level of phosphorus to occur and make one prone to dental cavities.

3. Vitamin B_1

   Large amounts of Vitamin B_1 can over a period of time cause a manganese deficiency. Initially, the taking of Vitamin B_1 *(thiamine)* will give you a burst of energy. The excess of this B vitamin may also cause a magnesium deficiency. Both manganese and magnesium are important, Eck says, in blood sugar problems. Because of this manganese/magnesium dificiency, Eck believes, they can develop over 70 different diseases . . . including diabetes.

4. IRON

   Iron supplements can cause a copper deficiency. When too much iron is taken, Eck states, you can cause extremely high blood pressure, migraine headaches, and arthritis. Many arthritics have iron deposits in the joints of the body. Eck also reveals:

   Over 51% of all the cases of heart disease have been found to have iron pigment deposits in the cardiac cells of the heart . . . largely from taking too much iron or an inability to properly metabolize iron.[1]

   To give iron to raise iron is to lower iron. This is true of every mineral. When you have an iron deficiency, you give manganese.

5. ZINC

   Zinc supplements can cause a copper deficiency resulting in a severe anemia. By causing a copper deficiency the following conditions may result—menstrual problems, prostrate disorders, allergies, arthritis and insomnia to name a few.

6. COPPER supplements can over a period of time result in a Vitamin C deficiency. Excessive copper can also cause a Vitamin B-1 and B-6 deficiency.

---

[1]Ibid.

Impotency and frigidity problems are intimately associated with mineral ratio imbalances caused by "stress," diabetes, hypothyroidism, adrenal insufficiency, etc.

The **seven** main indicators, from a hair analysis, of impotence in a male or frigidity in the female are:

1. A 3.3 to 1 or less of calcium to magnesium level indicates that the individual has sexual problems of impotence or frigidity. This inverted ratio is found particularly in diabetics.
2. Sodium/Potassium inversion. The normal ratio is 2.5 of sodium to 1 of potassium. If this is inverted (less than 1.8/1), it is an indicator of sexual problems.
3. Copper. A very high copper level is another indicator.
4. Zinc. Extremely low or high zincs can also indicate sexual dysfunction and be a cause of impotence or frigidity.
5. A Sodium/Magnesium ratio greater than 18/1.
6. A Sodium/Zinc ratio greater than 8/1.
7. A Calcium/Sodium ratio greater than 10/1.

In the problems of obesity (overweight), Dr. Eck breaks down individuals into broad categories such as:

> Fast oxidation
> Slow oxidation
> Mixed oxidation

There are 3 different ways people metabolize their food. Dr. Eck refers to this as _Oxidation_. Oxidation is the use or burning of foods to produce energy on a cellular level. Regarding oxidation, Dr. Eck identifies the categories and suggests:

1. They are so fast
they are breaking down their sugars very rapidly and they have a great increase in heat production as a result. They are the type of people who, when they eat, they perspire a lot. They are _"fast oxidizers."_ A _"fast oxidizer"_ is a person who has a hyperactive thyroid and hyperactive adrenal glands. They tend to have excessive energy levels due to the fast burning of foods, followed by exhaustion.

2. They are so _slow_

that they are metabolizing their foods very slowly. They are _"slow oxidizers."_ They have a hypoactive thyroid and hypoactive adrenal glands. Slow oxidizer's energy levels are usually low. This can be due to a number of factors such as the body's inability to completely break down the foods consumed when a HCl (Hydrochloric acid) deficiency is present. Low thyroid and adrenal activity also contributes to slow oxidation as well as toxic metal accumulation and dietary habits.

3. They are _mixed_ oxidizers

who may be fast in one glandular area and slow in another. They tend to have energy swings as well as mood swings. This is due to the _"seesaw"_ effect from fluctuating into fast and slow oxidation.

Both the fast and slow oxidizers are handling their foods the wrong way.

The Pill Destroys Sex Life Of Women

Dr. Eck believes that the Pill has destroyed the sex life of at least 10 million women.

The Pill creates a false pregnancy. The taking of a birth control pill raises the copper levels in the body. This creates a mineral imbalance which lowers your thyroid function as well as adrenal activity.

When a person has a low thyroid activity (hypothyroid), they don't have anywhere near the sex arousal . . . nor do they have a strong sex desire. They don't have the energy for it! Not only that, but the Pill brings with it menstrual period irregularities and menopausal disorders.

The male with high copper levels also develops a **slow** sexual arousal. Food that are high in copper include Brazil nuts, peanuts, sesame seeds, corn grits, broiled cod, baked flounder, broiled halibut, steamed lobster, pike and perch, ham, liver. Oysters are extremely high in copper. Just 1 cup of oysters (cooked, fried or raw) contains 59 milligrams of copper!

You also take copper into your body by drinking water coming through copper water pipes or cooking out of copper cookware.

Some women use a copper IUD birth control device. Because vaginal secretions are normally acid . . . that acidity leaches the copper off the coil and it goes into your system. Dr. Eck states that:

> *It is estimated that there is enough copper*
> *eroded from a coil in one year*
> *to actually cause susceptible individuals*
> *to become schizophrenic.*[1]

In a pregnant woman, the copper keeps building up during pregnancy. The fetus stores a large amount of copper that he gets from his mother's liver. This usually lasts the child for 12 years.

> *At the end of 12 years . . . if the child's copper level*
> *does not go down . . . you have females complaining of*
> *acne and adolescent problems, etc.*

If the mother cannot quickly unload the copper excess after pregnancy . . . she develops postpartum depression. Some women have become mentally unbalanced after giving birth. Paul Eck believes that copper excesses are the problem. Depending on the mineral imbalances of the individual, Eck uses either minerals or vitamins to unload the copper excesses. The hair analysis determines what supplements are needed.

What Results Can One Expect

Dr. Eck states that those who have a hair analysis and follow through on a personalized supplement program will experience symptomatic changes within two to three weeks. At least one year on supplements is needed to approach normalized mineral levels. Toxic metals and toxic minerals can be eliminated from the tissues in about 6 months.

They may experience periodic worsening of their general condition depending upon their findings. As an example, if a person has rheumatoid arthritis, many times within the first two weeks there may be a marked reduction in pain. However, if the individual has

---

[1]Schizophrenia is *a major mental disorder typically characterized by a separation between the thought processes and the emotions . . . a distortion of reality, accompanied by delusions and hallucinations.*

numerous heavy metal accumulations, the removal from tissues and joints of these toxic metals will trigger a temporary flare-up in their condition. This may occur several times throughout the program. Dr. Eck suggests that if this flare-up of symptoms becomes too severe, the individual should reduce or stop taking his supplements for a few days until the symptoms subside.

Permanents, tints, bleaching and coloring of hair does not make any insurmountable significant changes in hair analysis mineral readings. Some shampoos, hair treatments do affect mineral levels, however.

> Selsun Blue may cause an elevation in selenium levels.
> Head and Shoulders or Breck may result in elevated zinc.
> Grecian Formula or other darkening agents will many
>   times result in elevated lead levels. Lead acetate is used
>   in these products to blacken the hair.

Dr. Eck suggests that hair analysis retests should be done three months after the first test to check progress. If the individual is a *"mixed oxidizer"* or *"fast oxidizer,"* a retest is suggested in two months.

Dr. Eck says you cannot treat these people exactly the same as far as anything is concerned. You must take into consideration a broad classification of their oxidation types . . . preparing a program on that premise. You cannot give any one mineral for an obesity problem or any other problem. Hair analysis will determine what minerals are deficient and what minerals are in excess.

Paul Eck is very sold on proper hair analysis. In fact he is so sold on the necessity for hair analysis that he would not suggest any mode of treatment for any condition . . . to a physician . . . until a hair analysis of the patient has been made.

Hair analysis is becoming more and more popular. And there are quite a few hair analysis laboratories throughout the United States. Not all agree with Dr. Paul Eck's approach. In fact, he may be considered a maverick in the field. But his laboratory in Phoenix is kept very busy. It could be a sign that his customers are getting excellent results from his recommendations.[1]

---

[1]Dr. Paul Eck, Analytical Research Labs, Inc., 2338 West Royal Palm Road, Suite F, Phoenix, Arizona 85021.

FOR YOUR <u>LIFE</u> . . . KEEP INFORMED!

Now available! A quarterly Total Health Guide Newsletter to keep you up-to-date on the <u>very latest</u> of Medical/Nutritional Data! You owe it to yourself and to your loved ones . . . to be fully informed! Now! At last! You can have the <u>most current</u> information on diseases and their treatment . . . even before it is available to the general public! The information you receive may help save your life . . . or the life of a loved one!

<u>TWO</u> WAYS TO SUBSCRIBE

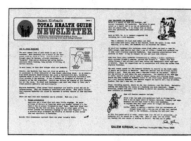

1. <u>Total Health Guide Newsletter</u>

Quarterly, for one year we will send you the 8-page Newsletter containing all the latest data on the major diseases. The Newsletter will present an unbiased report on both the Medical and Nutritional discoveries plus reports on their effectiveness and availability.

One Year: $25

2. Total Health Guide Newsletter
Plus
PERSONALIZED TYPEWRITTEN UPDATE

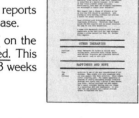

You will receive the quarterly 8-page Newsletter which reports the latest in Medical and Nutritional approaches to disease.

Plus! You will also receive a <u>TYPEWRITTEN REPORT</u> on the <u>specific disease in which you are personally interested</u>. This TYPEWRITTEN REPORT will be mailed to you within 3 weeks after you subscribe.

● You will also receive a <u>RING BINDER</u> to hold the Newsletters and Report. It will also contain a special unit to hold cassettes.

● Plus you will be sent the <u>cassette</u> . . .
   BALANCING YOUR EMOTIONS
   by Dr. Jonas Miller.

One Year: $50

SEE OTHER SIDE

SALEM KIRBAN, Inc., Kent Road, Huntingdon Valley, Pennsylvania 19006

- -

YES! I want to keep informed! Send me the Health Information Service I have checked below. My check is enclosed.

☐ 1 Year / $25
Total Health Newsletter

☐ 1 Year / $50 *(Fill in other side)*
Total Health Newsletter
Typewritten Health Report
(Includes Ring Binder/Cassette)

Mr./Mrs./Miss   (Please PRINT)

Address

City   State   ZIP

REQUEST For Personalized TYPEWRITTEN HEALTH UPDATE

If you are subscribing for Medical/Nutritional Health Information for One Year at $50, you are entitled to a Typewritten Health Update on one disease.

It is important you understand that we neither diagnose or prescribe. Therefore we **cannot** make personal recommendations to you. Only your physician can do this. What we do provide you is the very latest in both Medical and Nutritional information on the disease in which you are interested.

Each month we go through hundreds of publications, books and listen to both medical and nutritional seminar cassettes. We cull from all of this the data that is essential to the particular disease in which you are interested.

We would be happy to answer specific questions in this TYPEWRITTEN HEALTH UPDATE providing they are not in the realm of diagnosing or prescribing.

DISEASE I want Data on_____

MY QUESTIONS I particularly would like answered: *(Please PRINT)*

1. _____

_____

_____

2. _____

_____

_____

3. _____

_____

_____

4. _____

_____

_____

**FILL IN
RESPONSE FORM
ON
REVERSE SIDE
AND
MAIL WITH YOUR CHECK**

18

CARROTS, CAYENNE AND PARSLEY

VITAMIN C

Overcomes Poisons

Several tests done by medical nutritionists have shown that Vitamin C can help the body overcome foreign poisons (such as cadmium) that result from air, water and food pollution. Some suggest 1000 to 3000 milligrams daily.

Vitamin C is a good natural laxative, diluting bile and aiding in elimination. Several nutritionists recommend that the 1000 to 3000 milligrams of C be spread out over the day in units of 500 milligrams at a time . . . for better total absorption.

CAYENNE AND GARLIC

A Dynamic Duo

Many herbalists believe that a combination of Cayenne and Garlic can lower blood pressure, relieve indigestion, strengthen the heart and improve circulation. They recommend two capsules three times daily of Cayenne and Garlic combination. They also recommend that these capsules be taken with a large glass of water and preferably with meals.

Another herbalist combination capsule contains: Cayenne, Parsley, Ginger, Golden Seal Root and Garlic. They recommend taking two capsules with a large glass of water each morning and evening.

JUICE COMBINATIONS

**Keeps
Your
System
Flushing**

High blood pressure is reported by some to usually respond to a combination of carrot, celery and beet juice ... with a major portion of the 16 ounce drink made up of celery juice. Some nutritionists recommend drinking up to two quarts of this combination daily. At the same time as the liquid is taken, Cayenne-garlic capsules are also taken.

Other combinations include drinks of

> Carrot 10 ounces, spinach 6 ounces
> Carrot 10 ounces, beet 3 ounces,
>   cucumber 3 ounces
> Carrot 7 ounces, celery 4 ounces,
>   parsley 2 ounces, spinach 3 ounces

Many times people with high blood pressure eat a lot of salt and salty foods. Doctors urge patients to discontinue these. Also the drugs prescribed often deplete the potassium in one's body. Fruit juices are good sources of replenishing potassium ... naturally.

**Note
Please**

Anyone with High Blood Pressure should not start juice therapy without checking with their physician and should be carefully monitored.

DROPSY AND PARSLEY

**Parsley . . .
Life's
Forgotten
Food!**

The word, dropsy is from the Greek meaning *water*. Dropsy is not a disease, but rather a condition where fluid (*edema*) builds up in the tissues of the body. This is evidenced by swelling.

Dropsy can be caused by heart disease, kidney disease, cirrhosis of the liver and an excess of sodium retention.

You recall, earlier we discussed that those who suffer from High Blood Pressure are usually first given drugs which have a diuretic action. These *"fluid pills"* are designed to flush the sodium out through your urine. Drug diuretics have 15-20 side effects.

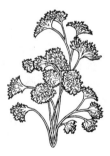

Parsley is nature's diuretic. Some nutritionists suggest for those who need a diuretic, the drinking daily of 2 quarts of parsley root. This is made either as a cold or warm tea concoction. The herb, in tea form, acts more rapidly than parsley capsules. Parsley is very high in Vitamin C and also has substantial amounts of calcium, magnesium, phosphorus, potassium and Vitamin A.

A Warning	**If fresh parsley is made into a juice . . . NEVER drink it by itself!** In this form it is highly concentrated and potent and will work very quickly on your system . . . throw out the poisons too fast and cause serious upsets.[1]
	Parsley juice (1 ounce) is best combined into a green drink made up of juice from beet tops, celery, endive, green beans and okra. Green drinks are an effective blood cleanser and blood builder.[2]
Garlic And Parsley	Some herbalists recommend taking two capsules of Garlic and Parsley with a large glass of water daily each morning and evening.

[1]Dr. John R. Christopher, A Sprig of Life, (Salt Lake City, Colorado: The Herbalist), March, 1978, pp. 15, 16.

[2]Salem Kirban, How Juices Restore Health Naturally, (Huntingdon Valley, Pennsylvania: Salem Kirban, Inc.), 1980, center color section. **For a copy of this book,** send $6 (includes postage) to: Salem Kirban, Inc., Kent Road, Huntingdon Valley, Pennsylvania 19006.

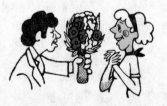

Next time don't give your sweetheart flowers. She can't eat them! Give her a bouquet of parsley and watch her face light up. Parsley is high in Vitamin A. It will make her skin lovelier and give her better vision to see the good points in you!

PARSNIP & PARSLEY SALAD
4 Servings

Never heard of a parsnip? Neither had I! Parsnips resemble carrots in shape. To bring out the best flavor in parsnips, store them for several weeks just a little above 32° in the frige. Parsnips discolor easily so do not peel them. Parsnips are rich in minerals.

Combine:

>   2 **cups shredded, raw parsnips**[1]
>   1 **cup fresh parsley finely cut**[2]
>   1 **tomato chopped fine**
>   2 **green onions chopped fine**
>   ¼ **cup quartered ripe olives**
>   1 **cup celery finely chopped**

Bathe this mixture in sufficient olive oil and toss lightly to mix. Add sufficient herb seasoning to taste plus:

>   **Juice of 1 lemon**

Parsnips are best purchased in the winter time after the first frost. This mellows and sweetens their flavor.

[1] *You may substitute salsify or oyster plant. However, salsify should be steamed first for about 10 minutes.*

[2] *If fresh parsley is not available, substitute ¼ cup dried parsley.*

For added joy, throw in some crushed garlic cloves and mix thoroughly with the olive oil.

PARSLEY LEMON BUTTER
4 Servings

Take:

>   ½ **cup butter**

and cream slightly softened butter, adding:

>   2 **tablespoons fresh lemon juice**

as it becomes pliable. Then add:

>   1 **teaspoon herb seasoning or sea salt**
>   **A pinch of cayenne pepper**
>   1 **tablespoon finely minced parsley**

Seasoned butters may be frozen for several weeks. However, they should not be refrigerated longer than 24 hours since the herbs deteriorate quickly.

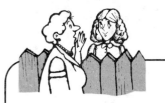

AUNT EFFIE . . .
Cousin Lulubelle is concerned about her facial blemishes!

Nature gives you the face you have at twenty; it is up to her to merit the face she has at forty! That woman is one of the Lee sisters and her first name is Ug. I never forget a face, but I'm willing to make an exception in her case. Cousin Lulubelle only seems to put on weight in certain places . . . pizza parlors, bakeries and ice cream shops.

Lulubelle oughta start eating that parsley and pushing the bacon and eggs aside if she's concerned about her face. I take a handful of fresh parsley, boil it in one pint of water for 10 minutes. Then I wash my face with this solution every morning upon arising and every evening before going to bed. It should be made fresh daily. I noticed an improvement in my complexion within one week!

If she takes a handful of parsley and boils it in one quart of water . . . making a broth . . . taking a few ounces at a time during the day, Lulubelle will find this will solve her "monthly" problems giving her smooth menstrual flow. And the same concoction is good for gout, arthritis, kidney stones, pinworms and gallbladder disorders. Tell her to take 2 cups daily before meals.

19

DIET CAN LOWER BLOOD PRESSURE

LOWER YOUR BLOOD PRESSURE WITH BETTER DIET

John M. Douglass, M.D., a Los Angeles, California internist took 32 persons with mild to severe High Blood Pressure and advised them to eat a 60 to 100% raw food diet. They were also told to eat salt sparingly. The results were heartwarming.[1]

A WELL BODY REBELS AT JUNK

A
Wise
Body

Once the body is detoxified it will no longer tolerate liquor and cigarettes. A well body will rebel against these poisons often causing nausea and vomiting. Some suggest there is a strong link between heavy drinking and hypertension.

Excess consumption of sugar is thought by many to be a major cause of hypertension. Meat-eating contributes to elevated blood pressure.

[1]Lower Your Blood Pressure with Better Diet, (Emmaus, Pennsylvania: Rodale Press), August, 1977, pp. 91-97.

Eliminating Meat

In a Harvard medical report, when meat was eliminated from one's diet, a fairly prompt response of lower blood pressure was noted. On the other hand, when meat was added to the diet, a fairly prompt elevation of blood pressure was noted.[1]

Sink Sugar!

Sugar has for a long time been associated with High Blood Pressure but the Harvard research team was surprised to learn that meat also is a contributory factor.

THE KILLER SALT

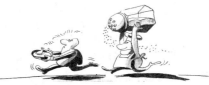

We Consume Far Too Much!

Most Americans consume about 20 times the necessary amount of salt daily!
Salt, or sodium chloride, is about 40% sodium and the main source of sodium in our diets.

One source of sodium that appears in many processed foods, sauces (like soy sauce) and canned soups is:

Monosodium glutamate (MSG)

MSG Another Culprit

Most doctors and nutritionists recommend that whenever you see Monosodium glutamate listed as an ingredient . . . that you avoid buying that product. This

[1]Frank M. Sacks, Bernard Rossner, Ph.D., Edward Kass, M.D., (American Journal of Epidemiology), November, 1974.

sodium compound is used as a *"flavor enhancer"* but simply adds to the over-supply of salt in our diet.

Causes Mood Changes

Salt can cause premenstrual tension, severe mood changes and stress. Salt can become an addiction . . . an addiction that strikes those who suffer most from its effects.

Salt Promotes Fluid Buildup!

Salt plays a major role in the cause of High Blood Pressure *(Hypertension)*. Hypertension is caused, in part, to some abnormality of the kidneys. The excessive salt we take into our body cannot be processed by the kidneys. There is a resultant fluid build-up which naturally, increases the volume of blood. Because of the higher blood volume, the rate of heartbeat increases. This, along with other factors increases blood pressure. While High Blood Pressure is not a disease . . . the resultant wear and tear from poor dietary habits can eventually lead to heart attacks, strokes, diabetes, kidney disease and other related ailments.[1]

[1]Marietta Whittlesey, Killer Salt, (New York: Bolder Books), 1977, pp. 46, 48.

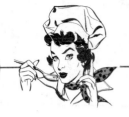

SALT ... THE HIDDEN KILLER

Big businesses thrive on our addiction to salt. If you wonder why you just can't stop eating some foods and *"empty calorie"* snacks, it is because of their high salt content.

Salt is called by many names and therefore is often confusing to the customer who seeks foods with a low salt content.

As an example, sodium nitrite and sodium nitrate are used extensively in the curing of meats and smoking of fish. (Nitrate is a source of nitrite). Sodium nitrite is present in all processed meat! This inlcudes cold cuts, hot dogs, bacon, ham, canned fish. It is also present, in the form of nitrite salts in our drinking water ... especially in areas where synthetic fertilizers are in use.

MSG/Monosodium Glutamate is sometimes called *"Chinese restaurant syndrome"* because it is used in large quantities in Chinese cooking to intensify the flavor of protein foods. One experiences headaches, dizziness, stomach pains and even fever if sensitive to this salt additive. You will find your canned soups and even bouillon cubes are full of it ... as well as many processed foods.

Sodium benzoate is another widely used salt preservative. It is often mixed in with salad dressings, relishes, baking power, baking soda and therefore finds its way in commercial bread.

Sodium sulfite is used to bleach fruits which are then colored to look more commercially attractive.

You will find salt in water softening devices. You can drink from 200 to 500 extra milligrams of sodium every day from such water!

A great many of the foods you buy in your supermarket are loaded with hidden salt! You must learn to read the labels. These should be dropped from your shopping list! Even your antacids are loaded with salt and many commercial laxatives!

The average American takes into his body 3-7 Grams of salt (sodium) and 6-28 Grams of sodium chloride each day!

There is a popular misconception that salt *improves* the taste of food. It does not! Foods have their own natural flavoring agents. Salt does **not** improve the taste of food – it masks it!

Your total salt intake should be kept at a level of from 1-4 Grams a day. For your health's sake ... it is preferable for you to strive for the lower range on the 1-4 scale aiming for a maximum of 1 Gram of salt per day! Your body will thank you ... with longer life!

Unfortunately, processed foods account for over 55% of the food Americans eat! Fresh garden peas, as an example, contain only 2 milligrams of sodium in a 3½ ounce serving. But that same portion of **canned** peas has 236 milligrams! And while canning increases the sodium content of vegetables dramatically . . . it decreases the amount of potassium in food. This is tragic . . . because potassium is beneficial in controlling high blood pressure.

Isn't this a good time . . . right this very minute . . . to go to your kitchen and **THROW AWAY the salt shaker!** For your life . . . and that of your loved ones . . . **do it right now!**

The following foods purchased from your food store are, for the most part, also very high in sodium.

1. Gravies and sauces
2. TV dinners, meals and entrees . . . frozen and canned
3. Pizzas
4. Pancake and waffle mixes
5. Lasagna and other pasta dishes
6. Macaroni, noodles, ravioli and spaghetti.
   (As an example, **just** an **8** ounce unit of spaghetti with meat sauce and meatballs can have as high as 1970 milligrams of sodium!)
7. Frozen pies and pastries
8. Canned, frozen and dehydrated soups and vegetables

Here's What Excessive Sodium Does To Your Body!

It whips the kidneys

Over the years of salt excesses, the kidneys suddenly fail to operate efficiently to get rid of enough sodium to maintain a healthy balance. The retained sodium holds water making the volume of blood to rise. Thus the blood vessels become water-logged. This water-logging makes them more sensitive to nerve stimulation . . . that causes them to contract.

Thus, more blood has to pass through the same ever-narrowing channels making the blood pressure increase. Because the heart has more blood to pump around the body . . . the heart rate also increases. This turns into a vicious cycle of **more blood** versus **narrower and contracting** blood vessels.

To add insult to injury . . . **stress** stimulates an adrenal-gland hormone, <u>aldosterone</u>. This signals the kidneys to hold on to sodium and water . . . and this <u>compounds</u> the problem!

Plus
the excess sodium in your system also increases the amount of <u>water</u> in and around the body tissues. Swelling occurs. Your doctor calls it *edema*. If the swelling reaches the heart . . . the heart cannot pump properly and <u>congestive heart failure occurs</u>.

People first notice swelling in their legs. This swelling interferes with the return of blood to the heart. This makes it difficult to walk and also encourages clots in the veins. Swelling can also occur in the brain. This can emotional problems including depression and irritability.

Just before the start of a menstrual period, the body has a tendency to retain sodium. This gives *premenstrual tension* and bloating with irritability and headache. For a woman to take salt during this time (when she craves it) makes the problem <u>worse</u>! The best advice is to be sure you have a <u>low-salt diet at least a week or 10 days before your period is due</u>.

In light of all this . . . **isn't it time for you to throw away your salt shaker** and **drastically reduce** your intake of processed foods! To do so . . . can add years to your life . . . and that of your loved ones!

SALT CONTENT of FOODS

Salt intake (in all its forms) should be limited to a total of 1-4 Grams a day. Those who already have an illness and those over 35 should keep their salt intake level preferably at 1 Gram per day.

A Milligram is one-thousandth of a Gram. Therefore, 1 Gram is 1000 Milligrams. The listings below give the Sodium (salt) content in Milligram units in those foods with **highest** salt content.

Those listings printed in **RED** indicate that just one serving exceeds the total recommended salt intake for the entire day! Salt intake daily should be limited to 1 Gram (1000 milligrams).

Food	Portion	Sodium (milligrams)
BEVERAGES		
Club Soda (Canada Dry)	8 oz.	60
Club Soda (Schweppes)	10 oz.	44
Coca Cola	8 oz.	20
Coffee and Tea		2
Diet Pepsi Cola	12 oz.	62
Tab	8 oz.	30
Diet 7-Up	12 oz.	48
Fresca, sugar free	12 oz.	61
A & W Root Beer	12 oz.	61
A & W Root Beer, sugar free	12 oz.	79
7-Up	12 oz.	32
Sprite	8 oz.	42
FRUIT DRINKS		
Lemon-lime and orange (Gatorade)	8 oz.	130
Orange Hi-C	6 oz.	58
VEGETABLE DRINKS		
Clamato	6 oz.	815
Tomato Cocktail (Firehouse Jubilee)	6 oz.	599
Vegetable Juice Cocktail (spicy hot, V-8)	6 oz.	569
(V-8 regular)	6 oz.	555
Tomato juice		
Libby	6 oz.	455
Del Monte	6 oz.	480
Stokely	8oz.	660

Food	Portion	Sodium (milligrams)
Milk Beverages		
Cocoa Mix	4 teaspoons	149
Cocoa Mix (Ovaltine)	1 oz.	183
(Nestle)	1 oz.	145
Buttermilk, from skim milk	1 cup	319
Condensed, sweetened	1 cup	343
Instant, non-fat, reconstituted	1 cup	322
Whole Milk	1 cup	122
Evaporated	1 cup	266
Milk Shake, thick chocolate	1 shake	333
Milk Shake, thick vanilla	1 shake	299
Malted Milk Shake	1 cup	215
Yogurt		
Low Fat Dannon	1 cup	235

(BREADS)

Food	Portion	Sodium (milligrams)
French, brown/serve		
Pepperidge Farm	2 oz.	415
Roman Meal	2 slices	320
Rye (Beefsteak)	2 slices	330
Pumpernickel	1 slice	182
Wheat		
Hollywood Light	2 slices	335
Pepperidge Farm	2 slices	405
Wonder	2 slices	375
Biscuits/Rolls		
Baking powder, dinner		
Tenderflake	2 biscuits	350
Buttermilk		
Big Country/Pillsbury	2 biscuits	720
Hungry Jack (extra rich)	2 biscuits	410
(Fluffy)	2 biscuits	605
Bisquick Mix	1/2 cup	700
Cornbread		
Ballard	1/8 package	695
Betty Crocker	1/12 package	300
Pepperidge Farm	1 oz. piece	518
Muffins		
Pepperidge Farm	1 muffin	633

Food	Portion	Sodium (milligrams)
Rolls		
Crescent, Pillsbury	2 rolls	760
Hoagie or Submarine roll	5 oz. roll	783
Crackers		
Graham	1 cracker	48
Rye	1 cracker	70
Saltine	2 crackers	70
Whole Wheat	1 cracker	30
Sesame sticks		
Pepperidge Farm	1 oz.	337
Stuffings		
Stuffing Bread	**8 oz. package**	**3021**
Stove Top Stuffing	1/6 package	490

BREAKFAST CEREALS

Food	Portion	Sodium (milligrams)
All-Bran	1 oz.	160
Alpha-Bits	1 cup	195
Bran Chex	2/3 cup	262
40% Bran	2/3 cup	251
100% Bran	1/2 cup	221
Raisin Bran	1/2 cup	209
Cheerios	1¼ cup	304
Corn Chex	1 cup	297
Corn Flakes	1 cup	256
Golden Grahams	1 oz.	345
Granola	1/4 cup	61
Grape Nuts	1 oz.	195
Kix	1½ cup	261
Life	2/3 cup	146
Post Toasties	1 oz.	305
Product 19	3/4 cup	175
Puffed Rice	2 cups	2
Raisins, Rice and Rye (Kellog's)	1 oz.	170
Rice Chex	1 cup	275
Rice Krinkles	1 oz.	185
Rice Krispies	1 oz.	340
Special K	1¼ cup	265
Sugar Frosted Flakes	1 oz.	230
Toasty O's	1 cup	280
Total	1 cup	359
Wheat Chex	2/3 cup	190
Wheaties	1 cup	355

Food	Portion	Sodium (milligrams)

BREAKFAST SWEETS

Food	Portion	Sodium
Coffee Cake	1 slice	152
Danish	1 roll	250
Doughnut		
Cake type	1 doughnut	160
Yeast leavened	1 doughnut	99
Sweet Rolls	1 roll	115
Toaster Pastry:		
Apple, frosted	1 pastry	324
Blueberry, frosted	1 pastry	242
Cinnamon, frosted	1 pastry	326
Strawberry	1 pastry	238

CHEESES

Food	Portion	Sodium
Natural:		
Blue	1 oz.	396
Brick	1 oz.	159
Brie	1 oz.	178
Camembert	1 oz.	238
Cheddar, regular	1 oz.	176
Colby	1 oz.	171
Cottage, regular, low fat	4 oz.	457
Cream	1 oz.	84
Edam	1 oz.	274
Feta	1 oz.	316
Gouda	1 oz.	232
Gruyere	1 oz.	95
Limburger	1 oz.	227
Monterey	1 oz.	152
Mozzarella	1 oz.	125
Muenster	1 oz.	178
Neufchatel	1 oz.	113
Parmesan	1 oz.	528
Provolone	1 oz.	248
Ricotta	1 oz.	125
Roquefort	1 oz.	513
Swiss	1 oz.	74
Tilsit	1 oz.	213
Pasteurized Processed Cheese:		
American	1 oz.	406
Swiss	1 oz.	388
Cheese Spread, American	1 oz.	381

Food	Portion	Sodium (milligrams)

CONDIMENTS

Food	Portion	Sodium (milligrams)
Bac O's	1 tablespoon	230
Baking powder	1 teaspoon	329
Baking soda	1 teaspoon	821
Catsup, regular	1 tablespoon	156
Garlic		
Powder	1 teaspoon	1
Salt	**1 teaspoon**	**1850**
Horse radish, prepared	1 tablespoon	198
Meat Tenderizer, regular	**1 teaspoon**	**1750**
MSG (monosodium glutamate)	1 teaspoon	492
Mustard, prepared	1 teaspoon	65
Olives		
Green	4 olives	323
Ripe, mission	3 olives	96
Onion		
Powder	1 teaspoon	1
Salt	**1 teaspoon**	**1620**
Pickles		
Bread and butter	2 slices	101
Dill	1 pickle	928
Sweet	1 pickle	128
Relish, sweet	1 tablespoon	124
Salt	**1 teaspoon**	**1938**
Sauces:		
A-1	1 tablespoon	275
Barbeque	1 tablespoon	130
Chili, regular	1 tablespoon	227
Cocktail	4 tablespoons	765
Soy	**1 tablespoon**	**1029**
Tabasco	1 teaspoon	24
Tartar	1 tablespoon	182
Teriyaki	1 tablespoon	690
Worcestershire	1 tablespoon	206

Food	Portion	Sodium (milligrams)

DESSERTS

Cakes, from mix
Angel food		
regular	1 slice	134
one step	1 slice	250
Devil's food	1 slice	402
Pound	1 slice	171
White	1 slice	238
Yellow	1 slice	242
Cheesecake	1 slice	350

Icings
Chocolate	1 cup	167
White	1 cup	156

Cookies
Brownies	1 brownie	69
Chocolate chip	4 cookies	140
Fig bars	2 bars	96
Ginger snaps	4 cookies	161
Shortbread	4 cookies	116
Sugar cookies	1 cookie	108
Molasses	3 cookies	125
Sandwich, chocolate or vanilla	4 cookies	193
Sunflower raisin		
Pepperidge Farm	3 cookies	236

Gelatins and Puddings
Custard, baked	1 cup	209
Puddings:		
Butterscotch:		
Regular, whole milk	½ cup	245
Instant, whole milk	½ cup	445
Ready-to-serve	1 can	290
Chocolate:		
Regular, whole milk	½ cup	195
Instant, whole milk	½ cup	470
Ready-to-serve	1 can	262
Vanilla:		
Regular, whole milk	½ cup	200
Instant, whole milk	½ cup	400
Ready-to-serve	½ cup	279
Tapioca, cooked	½ cup	130
Instant Jello	¼ package	420

Food	Portion	Sodium (milligrams)
Pies, frozen		
Apple	1 slice	208
Banana cream	1 slice	90
Bavarian cream	1 slice	78
Blueberry	1 slice	163
Cherry	1 slice	169
Chocolate cream	1 slice	107
Coconut cream	1 slice	104
Coconut custard	1 slice	194
Lemon cream	1 slice	92
Mince	1 slice	258
Peach	1 slice	169
Pecan	1 slice	241
Pumpkin	1 slice	169
Strawberry cream	1 slice	101

FAST FOODS

Food	Portion	Sodium (milligrams)
Big Mac	**average serving**	**1010**
Cheeseburger	average serving	709
Cheeseburger, double	**one**	**1414**
Cheeseburger, triple	**one**	**1848**
Chicken dinner	**1 portion**	**2243**
Fish sandwich	1 sandwich	882
Egg McMuffin	average serving	885
Hamburger:		
Regular	one	461
Double Beef Whopper	**one**	**1080**
Double Beef Whopper with Cheese	one	1535
Triple	one	1217
Hotcakes with butter & syrup	average serving	1070
French Fries	2.4 oz.	230
Onion Rings	2.7 oz.	450
Frankfurter	1 frankfurter	728
Pie, apple	3 oz. pie	398
Pie, cherry	3 oz. pie	427
Pizza, cheese	1/4 piece	599
Quarter Pounder	one average serving	735
Quarter Pounder with cheese	**average serving**	**1236**
Sausage	average serving	615
Scrambled eggs	average serving	205
Shake	1 shake	266

Food	Portion	Sodium (milligrams)

FISH

Food	Portion	Sodium (milligrams)
Bluefish, breaded, fried	3 oz.	123
Bonito, canned	3 oz.	437
Flounder, baked with butter	3 oz.	201
Haddock, breaded, fried	3 oz.	150
Halibut, broiled with butter	3 oz.	114
Herring, smoked	**3 oz.**	**5234**
Salmon, canned, salt added		
Pink	3 oz.	443
Red	3 oz.	329
Silver	3 oz.	298
Sardines, canned	3 oz.	552
Tuna, canned		
Light meat, chunk:		
Oil pack	3 oz.	303
Water pack	3 oz.	288
White meat (Albacore)		
Oil pack	3 oz.	384
Water pack	3 oz.	309
Shellfish		
Clams, hard, raw	3 oz.	174
Crab		
Canned, drained	3 oz.	425
Steamed	3 oz.	314
Lobster, boiled	3 oz.	212
Mussels, raw	3 oz.	243
Oysters		
Raw	3 oz.	113
Fried	3 oz.	174
Frozen	3 oz.	323
Scallops		
Raw	3 oz.	217
Steamed	3 oz.	225
Shrimp		
Raw	3 oz.	137
Fried	3 oz.	159
Canned	**3 oz.**	**1955**

Food	Portion	Sodium (milligrams)

FLOUR AND GRAINS

Food	Portion	Sodium (milligrams)
Bulgur, from hard red winter wheat	1 cup	621
Grits	1 oz.	658
Self-rising flour	**4 oz.**	**1520**
Brown rice	**3½ oz.**	**1360**
Minute Rice, flavored	1 serving	460
Spanish Rice	**1 cup**	**1480**

LEGUMES AND NUTS

Food	Portion	Sodium (milligrams)
Almonds, salted	1 cup	311
Beans, baked	1 cup	928
Beans, kidney (canned)	1 cup	844
Butter beans (Van Camp's)	1 cup	840
Lima beans, baby butter sauce frozen (Green Giant)	1 cup	885
Cashews, dry roasted	**1 cup**	**1200**
Peanuts		
dry roasted, salted	1 cup	986
roasted, salted	1 cup	601
Spanish, salted	1 cup	823
Soybeans (fermented/miso)		
Red	**1/4 cup**	**3708**
White	**1/4 cup**	**2126**
Peanut Butter	2 tablespoons	190

OILS AND SHORTENINGS

Food	Portion	Sodium (milligrams)
Butter, regular	1 tablespoon	116
Margarine, regular	1 tablespoon	140
Salad Dressing		
Blue cheese	1 tablespoon	153
French	1 tablespoon	214
Italian	1 tablespoon	116
Russian	1 tablespoon	133
Thousand Island	1 tablespoon	153
Mayonnaise	1 tablespoon	78

Food	Portion	Sodium (milligrams)
MEAT		
Beef		
Cooked, lean	3 oz.	55
Corned		
Cooked	3 oz.	802
Canned	3 oz.	893
Dried Chipped	**1 oz.**	**1219**
Lamb, lean	3 oz.	58
Pork:		
Cured:		
Bacon:		
Cooked	2 slices	274
Canadian	1 slice	394
Ham	**3 oz.**	**1114**
Salt pork, raw	1 oz.	399
Fresh cooked, lean	3 oz.	59
Veal, lean	3 oz.	69
Luncheon Meats		
Beer salami, beef	1 slice	56
Bologna:		
Beef	1 slice	220
Beef and pork	1 slice	224
Bratwurst, cooked	1 oz.	158
Braunschweiger	1 slice	324
Brotwurst	1 oz.	315
Chicken spread	1 oz.	115
Frankfurter	1 frankfurter	639
Ham:		
And cheese loaf	1 oz.	381
Chopped	1 slice	288
Deviled	1 oz.	253
Spread	1 oz.	258
Kielbasa	1 slice	280
Knockwurst	1 link	687
Lebanon bologna	1 slice	228
Liver cheese	1 slice	245
Liverwurst	1 oz.	330
Old fashioned loaf	1 slice	275
Olive loaf	1 slice	312
Pastrami	1 oz.	354
Pepperoni	1 slice	122
Pickle-and-pimiento loaf	1 oz.	394

Food	Portion	Sodium (milligrams)
Salami:		
Cooked:		
Beef	1 slice	255
Beef and pork	1 slice	234
Dry or hard, pork	1 slice	226
Sausage:		
Cooked:		
Pork	1 link	168
Pork and beef	1 patty	217
Smoked	1 link	264
Scrapple	1 slice	239
Turkey	2 oz.	498
Vienna sausage	1 link	152

Poultry and Game

Food	Portion	Sodium (milligrams)
Chicken, roasted:		
Breast with skin	½ breast	69
Drumstick with skin	1 drumstick	47
Products:		
Canned	5 oz. can	714
Frankfurter	1 frankfurter	617
Duck, roasted	1/2 duck	227
Goose, roasted	1/2 goose	543
Turkey, small, roasted		
Breast with skin	1/2 breast	182
Leg with skin	1 leg	195

SNACK FOODS

Food	Portion	Sodium (milligrams)
Breadsticks, no salt coating	10 8" sticks	350
Breadsticks, salt coated	10 8" sticks	837
Breakfast squares (General Mills)	2 bars	510
Bugles (General Mills)	1 oz.	335
Cheez Curls (Planters)	1 oz.	432
Chocolate Bar (Carnation Slender)	2 bars	358
Corn Chips (Planters)	1 oz.	220
Cupcake, chocolate (Hostess)	1 cupcake	250
Potato chips	10 chips	68
Potato chips (Planters)	1 oz.	210
Pretzels	1 Dutch type	268
Pretzels	10 rings	336
Pretzels	10 3" logs	840
Sticks, cheddar (Pepperidge Farm)	1 oz.	370

Food	Portion	Sodium (milligrams)
Sticks, whole wheat (Pepperidge Farm)	1 oz.	366
Tiger Tails (Hostess)	2 cakes	480
Twinkie (Hostess)	1 cake	190
Vanilla Bar (Carnation Slender)	2 bars	364

(SOUPS)

(**All** canned and dehydrated soups are high in sodium. Below sodium listings are only representative of the total available commercially prepared soups.)

Food	Portion	Sodium (milligrams)
Bean with bacon, condensed (Campbell's Manhandlers)	5½ oz.	1020
Bean with pork, condensed	11½ oz.	2627
Beef and country vegetables (Campbell's Chunky)	10¾ oz.	1035
Beef and noodles, condensed	5 oz.	910
Beef bouillon	1 cube	940
Beef broth and barley, cond.	5½ oz.	1100
Beef mushroom, condensed	5 oz.	1220
Beef noodle, condensed	1 cup	1041
Black bean, condensed	5½ oz.	1410
Burly vegetable, semi-condensed (Campbell's Soup for One)	7¾ oz.	1445
Chicken gumbo, condensed	1 cup	2160
Chicken noodle, condensed	1 cup	1107
Chicken noodle, dehydrated	2 oz. package	2438
Chicken rice, condensed	1 cup	814
Clam chowder, Manhattan, cond.	1 cup	1808
Minestrone, condensed	1 cup	992
Mushroom, condensed	1 cup	1031
Onion, condensed	1 cup	1407
Pea, green, condensed	1 cup	987
Scotch broth, condensed (Campbell's Manhandlers)	5 oz.	1050
Sirloin burger (Campbell's Chunky)	10¾ oz.	1140
Tomato, condensed	1 cup	872
*Vegetable, condensed	1 cup	823
Vegetable beef, condensed	1 cup	957

---

*While all grocery-store-purchased soups are high in sodium . . . the dehydrated variety are usually higher than the condensed variety. As an example . . . one cup of vegetable soup (condensed) has 823 milligrams of sodium. But one cup of vegetable soup (dehydrated) has a much higher 1146 milligrams of sodium.

Food	Portion	Sodium (milligrams)
VEGETABLES		
Asparagus, canned	4 spears	298
Beans, canned		
Italian	1 cup	913
Lima	1 cup	456
Snap	1 cup	326
Beets, canned		
Sliced	1 cup	479
Pickled	1 cup	330
Broccoli, frozen with cheese sauce	3.3 oz.	440
Brussels Sprouts, frozen in butter sauce	3.3 oz.	421
Carrots, frozen		
with brown sugar glaze	3.3 oz.	500
in butter sauce	3.3 oz.	350
Cauliflower, frozen with cheese sauce	3 oz.	325
Corn, canned		
cream style, regular	1 cup	671
vacuum pack	1 cup	577
whole kernel, regular	1 cup	384
Mushrooms, canned	2 oz.	242
Peas, frozen, regular	3 oz.	80
in butter sauce	3.3 oz.	402
in cream sauce	2.6 oz.	420
with mushrooms	3.3 oz.	240
Peas, canned, regular	1 cup	493
Potatoes, frozen		
Salted, french fries	2.5 oz.	270
Potatoes, canned	1 cup	753
Potatoes, instant, reconstituted	1 cup	485
Potatoes, mashed, milk & salt	1 cup	632
Potatoes, Au gratin	**1 cup**	**1095**
Saurkraut, canned	**1 cup**	**1554**
Spinach, frozen, creamed	3 oz.	280
canned, regular	1 cup	910
Spinach, New Zealand	1 lb.	721
Squash, canned, Summer	1 cup	785
Tomatoes, canned		
Whole	1 cup	390
Stewed	1 cup	584
Tomato Juice, regular	1 cup	878

Food	Portion	Sodium (milligrams)
Tomato paste	1 cup	77
Tomato puree, canned	**16 oz.**	**1809**
Tomato sauce	**1 cup**	**1498**
Vegetable juice cocktail	1 cup	887
Chinese frozen, (La Choy)		**1552**
Japanese frozen (La Choy)		**1224**
Stir Fry vegetables	3.3 oz.	500
Salads		
Bean, canned	1/2 cup	537
Carrot-raisin	1/2 cup	97
Cole Slaw	1/2 cup	68
Macaroni	2/3 cup	676
Potato	1/2 cup	625

(NONPRESCRIPTION DRUGS) Sodium content per dose

Aspirin	49
Antacid, analgesic:	
Bromo Seltzer	717
Alka-Seltzer (blue box)	521
Antacid, laxative:	
Sal Hepatica	**1000**
Antacids:	
Rolaids	53
Soda Mint	89
Alka-Seltzer Antacid (gold box)	276
Brioschi	710

(Vitamin C in <u>sodium ascorbate</u> form is high in sodium. Natural Vitamin C <u>(ascorbic acid)</u> is okay!)

Laxatives:	
Metamucil Instant	250
Fleet's Enema	250
Sleep-Aids:	
Miles Nervine	544
Antacid, suspensions	
Milk of Magnesia	10
Maalox	50
Mylanta I	76
Mylanta II	160
DiGel	170
Titralac	220

Exercise Can Lower Blood Pressure

About 54 seconds a day is all it takes to lower your blood pressure, according to Broino Kiveloff, M.D. Dr. Kiveloff is Director of physical medicine and rehabilitation at the New York Infirmary. He suggests that isometrics, a form of exercise, is beneficial in lowering blood pressure.

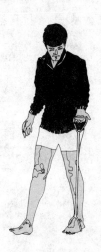

Isometrics is a method of physical exercise in which one set of muscles is tensed for a period of seconds, in opposition to another set of muscles or to an immovable object.

In the May, 1978 issue of Prevention Magazine, Dr. Kiveloff outlined his program of exercise.

He offers several initial guidelines:

1. Maintain *normal* breathing.
2. Spend only 6 seconds per exercise.
3. Count out loud one to six while doing the exercise. This helps you keep track of time and also helps you breathe properly.

To perform the exercises:

1. Stand in a relaxed position.
2. Tense all your muscles as tightly as possible for 6 seconds (while breathing normally and counting out loud).
3. Rest several seconds.
4. Repeat exercise twice more.
5. Do this three times a day.
6. Do not clench fists, bend elbows or other joints. Tighten your muscles in the position they assume with the least amount of motion.

Dr. Kiveloff reports that in his experience, it takes from 5-8 weeks of doing the exercise for the blood pressure to drop significantly. And the results will last if you keep up the program.

20

A SURVIVOR OR A STATISTIC

NOISE AND HIGH BLOOD PRESSURE

**Throw
Out Those
Rock Records!**

A noisy environment can lead to High Blood Pressure. Numerous tests have come up with this conclusion.

Investigators went into a Volvo automobile factory in Sweden to check for the effect of industrial noise on workers' blood pressure. One group consisted of men with noise-induced hearing loss, the other of men with normal hearing.

**Hearing Loss
And
High Blood
Pressure**

All 44 of the men with hearing loss turned out to have significantly higher blood pressure than the 74 men with normal hearing. The conclusion of these investigators was that:

> . . . *prolonged exposure
> to a stressful stimulus
> may have caused
> repeated rises in blood pressure
> leading to circulatory adaptations
> and a permanent rise in blood pressure.*[1]

Why does noise affect blood pressure? Noise stimulates the nervous system. This activates the adrenal glands. They secrete

---

[1]Noise, Sleep and Your Blood Pressure, (Emmaus, Pennsylvania: Rodale Press), October, 1977, pp. 110, 111 (from *Lancet*, January 8, 1977).

a hormone (*Adrenaline*) which not only affects the function of the heart but also increases the release of free fatty acids in the blood. Cholesterol is one of these fatty acids.

Cortisol (*another adrenal hormone*) is also released. There is a belief that this slows down the liver's ability to detoxify cancer-causing chemicals.

A SURVIVOR OR STATISTIC

**Time
For A
Change!**

High Blood Pressure has been called *The Silent Destroyer*. While there are no warning signs, there are areas in diet and living habits that can avoid or minimize the tendency towards rising blood pressure.

How often you have heard the saying:

*An ounce of prevention
is worth
a pound of cure.*

High Blood Pressure is a symptom of a so-called modern, progressive society. Perhaps it is time we get back to some old-fashioned basics in lifestyle and in eating habits. A positive mental approach and a **resolve** to make some changes in your life pattern are essential if you desire to be a survivor, rather than a statistic!

Use this ORDER FORM to order additional copies of

**The
MEDICAL Approach
Versus
NUTRITIONAL Approach
To
HIGH BLOOD PRESSURE**
by Salem Kirban

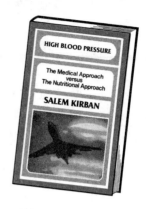

Your loved ones and friends will find
this book invaluable! Why not give this
excellent book to those who want hon-
est answers to their problems.

QUANTITY PRICES:

1 copy: $5.00

**3 copies: $12 (You save $3)
5 copies: $20 (You save $5)**

ORDER FORM

**Salem Kirban, Inc.
Kent Road
Huntingdon Valley, Pennsylvania 19006**

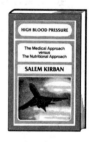

Enclosed find $ _____ (plus $1 postage) for _____ copies of

**The MEDICAL Approach Versus The NUTRITIONAL
Approach to HIGH BLOOD PRESSURE**
by Salem Kirban

Name_____
     Mr./Mrs./Miss   (Please PRINT)

Street_____

City_____

State_____Zip Code_____

KEY TO READING FOOD CHARTS

The Food Charts on the following pages are divided into 11 categories:

1. Meat and Poultry
2. Fish
3. Eggs
4. Milk and Dairy Products
5. Vegetables and Vegetable Products
6. Dry Beans, Peas and Nuts
7. Fruit and Fruit Products
8. Cereal, Grains and Grain Products
9. Fats and Oils
10. Sugars, Sweets and Syrups
11. Food Juices, Beverages

Bold Face Numerals
For each food listed, the highest mineral or vitamin content is printed in a bold face. As an example, in Chart 1 of Meat and Poultry . . . under Beef . . . the Chuck, boneless is highest in Potassium. Therefore the **354** milligrams is printed in **bold face type.**

Asterisks (*)
Some foods are preceded by an asterisk (*). These are foods which should **not** be included in your diet. There are unclean foods. But more important, they release their energy too quickly for the body to make use of them. They digest so fast that you cannot use the proteins, which turn into urea and dump into the bloodstream so fast that the kidneys cannot eliminate them. A urea build-up in the body ensues and excessive urea leads to many health problems.

High Stress Foods
The Food Charts indicate which foods are High Stress Foods. High Stress Foods should **not** be a major part of your food intake. You will find that eating too many High Stress Foods robs your body of energy. Plan your meals around **low stress** foods for better health.

Low Stress Foods
Low Stress Foods digest easily and quickly. They leave very little residue for the liver to detoxify. And, they do not cause toxic build-up in the colon or vascular system. Because Low Stress Foods are more easily digested, the (a) offer their energy more readily to the body and (b) conserve energy that would otherwise be used in trying to digest High Stress Foods. Therefore, this energy can be used to increase energy reserves and increase endurance.

1. MEAT and POULTRY

Food	Food Energy Calories	Basic Food Elements			MINERALS (Milligrams)								VITAMINS	
		Protein	Fat	Carbohydrates	Calcium	Phosphorus	Iron	Sodium	Potassium	Magnesium	Manganese	Zinc	Vitamin A	Vitamin C
HIGH STRESS														
Beef														
Chuck, boneless	257	18.7	19.6	0	11	168.2	2.8	64.9	354	18.5			39.6	
Corned hash, canned	199	8.9	14.6	8.09	26.1	69.6	1.2	540	200				tr	
Ground	263	25.6	17.0	0	7.1	220	3.9	47	449.2	21.2				
Heart	108	16.9	3.7	0.7	9	203	4.6	90	160	4.6			30	6
Kidney	141	15.0	8.1	0.9	9	221	7.9	245	231	18			1150	13
Liver, beef	136	19.7	3.2	6.0	7	358	6.6	86	325	21			43,900	31
Liver, calf	141	19.0	4.9	4.0	6	343	10.6	131	436	24			22,500	36
Lungs	96	17.6	2.3	0		216								
Porterhouse	242	25.4	14.7	0	11	183	3.8	52	398	20			617.2	
Potpie	195	7.3	11.2	16.3	6.2	48	1.5	366	93					
Ribs, lean	171	26.8	6.3	0	9.8	205	3.4	41.5	412.4	22.0				
Round, bottom	238	35.5	9.5	0	12.3	228	5.3	44.7	484	24.6				
Rump	235	32	10.9	0	8.8	197.5	4.8	53.8	386.2	20.0				
Sweetbreads	184	15.2	13.2	0	10	400	1.2	96	360				17	44
T-bone, broiled	247	25.3	15.5	0	10.5	181.1	3.8	51.6	398	20.0				
Tongue	208	16.4	15.1	0.4	8.1	182.3	2.1	73.3	197.4	16				
Brains	125	10.4	8.6	0.8	10.6	311.8	2.4	124.7	218.8					17.6

Food	Food Energy Calories	Protein	Fat	Carbohydrates	Calcium	Phosphorus	Iron	Sodium	Potassium	Magnesium	Manganese	Zinc	Vitamin A	Vitamin C
		Basic Food Elements					MINERALS (Milligrams)						VITAMINS	
Chicken														
Boned, canned	178	20.4	10.0	0.2	14	149	1.8		138					
Breast, fryer	104	23.3	0.5	0	14	212	1.1	90	370					
Broiler	151	20.2	7.2	0	14	200	1.5	78	320					
Gizzard	113	20.1	2.7	0.7	9.9	105.1	2.9	65.1	240.4					
Leg, fryer	112	20.5	2.7	0	15	188	1.8	79	325					
Liver	141	22.1	4.0	2.6	16	240	7.4	76.6	188				32,200	20
Potpie	198	8.3	10.4	17.4	16.4	101.7	1.0	411	153				123.3	5.2
Roaster	200	20.2	2.6	0	14	200	1.5	78	320					
Lamb														
Blade chop, lean	34	22.8	27	0	10	179	1.5	70	290	22				
Leg, lean, roasted	192	28.6	7.7	0	12	237	2.2	70	290	22				
Liver	261	32.3	12.4	2.8	16	572	17.9	85	331	20			74,500	36
Loin, lean	188	28.2	7.8	0	12	219	2.0	70	290	20				
*Pork														
Blade, lean	245	27.6	14.1	0	12	287	3.5	65	390	20				
Lion chop, broiled	418	23.5	35.2	0	10	256	3.2	65	390	22				
Picnic ham	323	22.4	25.2	0	10	182	2.9		25					
Spare ribs	440	28.8	38.9	0	9	121	2.6	65	390					
Turkey														
Roasted	200	30.9	7.6	0	30	400	5.1	129.5	367	28			10	
Veal														
Cutlet	277	33.2	15.0	0	10	288	4.2	54	527	23				
Loin chop	421	22.7	35.9	0	6	187	2.9	44	314	16				
Sirloin	274	23.9	19.1	0	8	221	3.0	53	476	19				

2. FISH

Food	Food Energy Calories	Basic Food Elements					MINERALS (Milligrams)							VITAMINS	
		Protein	Fat	Carbo-hydrates	Cal-cium	Phos-phorus	Iron	So-dium	Potas-sium	Magne-sium	Manga-nese	Zinc	Vitamin A	Vitamin C
HIGH STRESS														
Anchovy, canned	175	19.2	10	trace	166.6	208.2								
Bass, striped	105	18.9	2.7	0		212								
Caviar, pressed, canned	320	34	17	5				22	18					
*Clams														
Hard, raw	80	11.1	0.9	5.9	69	151	7.5	205	311			1.5		
Soft, raw	82	14.0	1.9	1.3		183	3.4	36	235			1.5		
Clam chowder	30	0.9	1.0	4.1	17.5	21.5	0.4	414						2
Cod	78	17.6	0.3	0	10	194	0.4	70	382	28				2
*Crab, steamed	93	17.3	1.9	0.5	43	175	0.8			34			2170	
*Fish cakes	172	14.7	8.0	9.3	—	195	—		—	—			—	
Flounder	68	14.9	0.5	0	61	195	0.8	56	366	30		0.7		
*Frog legs	73	16.4	0.3	0	18	147	1.5							
Halibut	100	20.9	1.2	0	13	211	0.7	54	449				440	
*Lobster														
Meat only	91	16.9	1.9	0.5	29.1	183	0.6							
Newburg	194	18.5	10.6	5.1	87	192	0.9	229	171					
*Oysters														
Eastern, raw	66	8.4	1.8	3.4	94	143	5.5	73	121	32		74.7	310	
Western, raw	91	10.6	2.2	6.4	85	153	7.2							30

Food	Food Energy Calories	Basic Food Elements			MINERALS (Milligrams)								VITAMINS	
		Protein	Fat	Carbohydrates	Calcium	Phosphorus	Iron	Sodium	Potassium	Magnesium	Manganese	Zinc	Vitamin A	Vitamin C
Salmon														
Atlantic	217	22.5	13.4	0	79	**186**	0.9							9
Chinook	222	19.1	15.6	0		301		45	**399**				310	
Pink	119	20.0	3.7	0				64	**306**					
Sardines														
Atlantic, in oil	311	20.6	24.4	0.6	354	434	3.5	510	**560**				180	
Pacific, in brine/mustard	196	18.8	12.0	1.7	303	354	5.2	**760**	260				30	
*Scallops, steamed	112	23.2	1.4		115	338	3.0	265	**476**					
*Shrimp	91	18.8	0.8	1.5	63	166	1.6	140	220	42		1.5		
Trout														
Brook	101	19.2	2.1	0		266								
Rainbow	195	21.5	11.4	0	—	—	—	—	—				—	—
*Tuna														
Canned in oil	288	24.2	20.5	0	6	294	1.1	**800**	301			1.0	90	
Canned in water	127	28.0	0.8	0	16	190	1.6	41	**279**					

3. EGGS

Food	Food Energy Calories	Basic Food Elements			MINERALS (Milligrams)								VITAMINS	
		Protein	Fat	Carbohydrates	Calcium	Phosphorus	Iron	Sodium	Potassium	Magnesium	Manganese	Zinc	Vitamin A	Vitamin C
Chicken Eggs														
whole, 1 medium	80	6	6	4	27	**205**	1.1	59	62	11		1.0	590	
Yolk	60	7	8	1	51	**205**	1.1	45	43	10.6		1.0	690	

4. MILK and DAIRY PRODUCTS

Food	Food Energy Calories	Basic Food Elements			MINERALS (Milligrams)								VITAMINS	
		Protein	Fat	Carbohydrates	Calcium	Phosphorus	Iron	Sodium	Potassium	Magnesium	Manganese	Zinc	Vitamin A	Vitamin C
low stress														
Buttermilk														
from skim milk	36.9	3.7	trace	4.9	121.4	95	0.04	130	**140**	14			4.1	0.8
Cheese														
American cheddar	398	25.0	32.2	2.1	**750**	478	1.0	700	82	45		4.0	1310	
Cottage, creamed	106	13.6	4.2	2.9	94	152	0.3	**229**	85				170	
Cottage, uncreamed	86	17.0	0.3	2.7	90	175	0.4	**290**	72				10	
Parmesan	393	35.7	26.1	2.9	**1142.4**	781.8	0.4	731.8	149.9	46.4			1071	
Swiss	371	27.5	27.9	1.8	**924.6**	564	1.1	710	104	43			**1449**	
Milk, skim non-instant	363	35.9	.8	52.3	1308	1016	.6	532	**1745**	143		.04	30	7
Sour cream	188	2.6	17.8	3.3	**102.3**	75.9		39.6	55.3	10			**759**	0.8
Yogurt	62	3.0	3.4	4.9	111.1	86.9		47.2	**132**				139.4	0.8
HIGH STRESS														
Butter														
salted	706	.6	81.	.4	20	16		**987**		2		0.1	**3300**	
unsalted	715	.6	82.	.4	**20**	16		8	9				**3350**	
Cheese														
American processed	370	23.2	30	1.9	697.1	478	0.9	**1136**	80	45		4.0	**1219**	
Margarine	719	0.6	80.7	0.4	20.0	16.1		**985**	23			0.2	**3310**	
Milk														
whole	65	3.5	3.5	4.9	117.7	92.8	0.04	49.9	**143.9**	13		0.4	143	1.1
goat's	67	3.2	4.	4.6	129	106	.1	34	**180**	17			160	1

5. VEGETABLES and VEGETABLE PRODUCTS

Food	Food Energy Calories	Protein	Fat	Carbo-hydrates	Cal-cium	Phos-phorus	Iron	So-dium	Potas-sium	Magne-sium	Manga-nese	Zinc	Vitamin A	Vitamin C
low stress														
Artichoke, globe	7	2.9	0.2	10.6	51	88	1.3	43	**430**				160	12
Asparagus, boiled	20	2.2	0.2	3.6	21	50	0.6	1	**183**	20			**900**	26
Beets, cooked	32	1.1	0.1	7.2	14	23	0.5	43	208	15			20	6
Beet Greens, raw	24	2.2	.3	4.6	119	40	3.3	130	**570**	106			**6100**	30
Broccoli, boiled	26	3.1	0.3	4.5	88	62	0.8	10	267	24			**2500**	90
Brussel Sprouts, boiled	36	4.2	0.4	6.4	32	72	1.1	10	273	29			520	87
Cabbage														
Chinese, raw	14	1.2	0.1	3.0	43	40	0.6	23	253	14			150	25
Headed	24	1.3	0.2	5.4	49	29	0.4	20	233	13		0.4	130	47
Red, raw	31	2.0	0.2	6.9	42	35	0.8	26	268				40	61
Carrots, raw	42	1.1	0.2	9.7	37	36	0.7	47	341	23		0.4	**11,000**	8
Cauliflower, boiled	22	2.3	0.2	4.1	21	42	0.7	9	206				60	55
Celery, raw	17	0.9	0.1	3.9	39	28	0.3	126	341	22			240	9
Collards, leaves, raw	45	4.8	0.8	7.5	250	82	1.5		**450**	57	0.16		**9300**	152
Corn, boiled	83	3.2	1.0	18.8	3	89	0.6		165	48			400	7
Cucumbers, with skin	15	0.9	0.1	3.4	25	27	1.1	6	160	11		0.4	250	11
Dandelion greens, raw	45	2.7	.7	9.2	187	66	3.1	76	397	36			**14,000**	35
Eggplant	19	1.0	.2	4.1	11	21	.6	1	150	16			10	3
Endive, raw	20	1.7	0.1	4.1	81	54	1.7	14	294	10			**3300**	10
Escarole, raw	20	1.7	0.1	4.1	81	54	1.7	14	294				**3300**	10
Garlic, raw	137	6.2	0.2	30.8	29	202	1.5	19	529					15

Food	Basic Food Elements				Calcium	Phosphorus	MINERALS (Milligrams)							VITAMINS	
	Food Energy Calories	Protein	Fat	Carbohydrates			Iron	Sodium	Potassium	Magnesium	Manganese	Zinc		Vitamin A	Vitamin C
Kale, cooked	28	3.2	0.7	4.0	134	46	1.2	43	221	37(raw)			7400	62
Kohlrabi, raw	29	2.0	0.1	6.6	41	51	0.5	8	372	37	0.11		20	66
Lentils														
cooked	106	7.8	—	19.3	25	119	2.1	—	249				20	
raw	340	24.7	1.11	60.1	79	377	6.8	30	790	80			60	
Lettuce														
Loose leaf	18	1.3	0.3	3.5	68	25	1.4	9	264			0.4	1900	18
Romaine	18	1.3	0.3	3.5	68	25	1.4	9	264	11			1900	18
Mushrooms	28	2.7	0.3	4.4	6	116	0.8	15	414	13				3
Okra	36	2.4	0.3	7.6	92	51	0.6	3	249	41	0.08	0.28	520	31
Olives														
black	86	0.6	9.4	1.5	49.7		0.8	381	15.9				30.8	
green	185	1.0	20	3.0	105	15	1.5	750	25	22		6	40	
Onions														
dry	38	1.5	0.1	8.7	27	36	0.5	10	157	12		0.3	40	10
young green, raw	36	1.5	0.2	8.2	51	39	1.0	5	231			0.3	2000	32
Parsley	44	3.6	0.6	8.5	203	63	6.2	45	727	41	0.9		8500	172
Parsnips, raw	76	1.7	0.5	17.5	50	77	0.7	12	541	32	0.03		30	16
Peas, boiled	71	5.4	0.4	12.1	23	99	1.8	1	196	35(raw)		0.7	540	20

Food	Basic Food Elements				MINERALS (Milligrams)								VITAMINS	
	Food Energy Calories	Protein	Fat	Carbohydrates	Calcium	Phosphorus	Iron	Sodium	Potassium	Magnesium	Manganese	Zinc	Vitamin A	Vitamin C
Peppers														
red, raw	31	1.4	0.3	7.1	13	**30**	0.6	13	**213**	18			**4450**	204
sweet green, raw	22	1.2	0.2	4.8	9	22	0.7						**420**	128
Pickles, dill	11	0.7	0.2	2.2	26	21	1.0	**1428**	200	12			100	6
Radish	17	1.0	0.1	3.6	30	31	1.0	18	**322**	15			10	26
Rutabaga	46	1.1	0.1	11.0	66	39	0.4	5	**239**	15			**580**	43
Salad with raw														
lettuce	28	0.2	0.05	0.6	11.6	4.2	0.24	1.5	44	(1.9)			323	3
carrots	28	0.2	0.03	1.6	6.3	6.0	0.12	8.0	58	3.9		0.07	1870	1.4
green pepper	28	0.2	0.03	0.8	1.5	3.7	0.12	2.2	36	3.0			70	21.7
onion	28	0.3	0.02	1.5	4.6	6.0	0.08	1.7	27	2.0		0.05	7	1.7
spinach	28	0.5	0.05	0.7	15.8	8.7	0.53	12.1	80	15.0		0.14	1377	8.7
radish	28	0.2	0.02	0.6	5.0	5.2	0.17	3.0	54	2.5			2	4.3
TOTALS		1.6	0.2	5.8	44.8	33.8	1.26	28.5	**299**	28.3		0.26	**3649**	40.8
Salad with raw														
carrot	27	0.3	0.05	2.4	9.2	9.0	0.18	11.8	85.2	5.8		0.1	2750	2
celery	27	0.2	0.02	1.0	9.8	7.0	0.08	31.5	85.2	5.5			60	2.2
spinach	27	0.8	0.08	1.1	23.2	12.8	0.78	17.8	117.5	22.0		0.2	2025	12.7
tomato	27	0.3	0.05	1.2	3.2	6.8	0.12	0.8	61.0	3.5		0.05	225	5.8
TOTALS		1.6	0.2	5.7	45.4	35.6	1.16	61.9	**348.9**	36.8		0.35	**5060**	22.7

Food	Food Energy Calories	Basic Food Elements								MINERALS (Milligrams)			VITAMINS	
		Protein	Fat	Carbo-hydrates	Cal-cium	Phos-phorus	Iron	So-dium	Potas-sium	Magne-sium	Manga-nese	Zinc	Vitamin A	Vitamin C
low stress														
Salad with steamed														
carrots	29	0.2	0.05	1.8	8.2	7.8	0.15	8.2	55.5			0.08	2625	1.5
green beans	29	0.4	tr.	1.4	12.6	9.2	0.15	1	37.8	8		0.08	136	3
okra	29	0.5	0.075	1.5	23	10.2	0.12	0.5	43.5	10.2			122.5	5
beets	29	0.3	0.025	1.8	3.5	5.8	0.12	10.8	52	3.8			5	1.5
TOTALS	29	1.4	0.15	6.5	47.3	33	0.54	20.5	188.8	22		0.16	2888.5	11
Sauerkraut	18	1.0	0.2	4.0	36	18	0.5	747	140				50	14
Soup														
Onion	26	2.2	1.05	1.9	11.5	11.5	0.2	434						
Vegetable	32	1.3	0.6	5.2	7.5	17.5	0.45	284					1264	
Squash														
Summer	19	1.1	0.1	4.2	28	29	0.4	1	202	16			410	22
Winter	50	1.4	0.3	12.4	22	38	0.6	1	369	17			3700	13
Sweet potato														
Candied	168	1.3	3.3	34.2	37	43	0.9	42	190				6300	10
Raw	114	1.7	0.4	26.3	32	47	0.7	10	243	31			8800	21
Swiss chard	25	2.4	0.3	4.6	88	39	3.2	147	550	65			6500	32
Turnips	30	1.0	0.2	6.6	39	30	0.5	49	268	20				36
Turnip greens, raw	28	3.0	.3	5.0	246	58	1.8	236	243	58			7600	139
Watercress, raw	19	2.2	.3	3.0	151	54	1.7	5.2	282	20			4900	79
Yams	101	2.1	0.2	23.2	20	69	0.6		600					9

Food	Basic Food Elements				Minerals (Milligrams)								Vitamins	
	Food Energy Calories	Protein	Fat	Carbohydrates	Calcium	Phosphorus	Iron	Sodium	Potassium	Magnesium	Manganese	Zinc	Vitamin A	Vitamin C
Horseradish, prepared	38	1.3	0.2	9.6	61.1	32	0.9	96	290.3					1.1
Lettuce														
Butterhead	14	1.2	0.2	2.5	35	26	2.0	9	264	11			970	8
Crisphead (iceberg)	14	1.2	0.2	2.5	35	26	2.0	9	264	11	0.4		970	8
Mustard greens	31	3.0	.5	5.6	183	50	3.0	32	377	27			7000	97
Potatoes														
Baked without skin	95	2.6	0.1	21.1	9	65	0.7	4	503	22(raw)				20
French-fried	771	12.7	29.5	118.4	32	304	6.4	14	2,295					41
Mashed	340	7.7	.5	77.6	73	177	3.2	358	1,039				140	29
Spinach	26	3.2	0.3	4.3	93	51	3.1	71	470	88	0.8		8100	51
Spinach, New Zealand	19	2.2	.3	3.1	58	46	2.6	159	795	166	1.6		4300	30
Tomatoes	22	1.1	0.2	4.7	13	27	0.5	3	244	14	0.2		900	23
Tomato catsup	106	2.0	0.4	25.4	22	50	0.8	1042	363	21			1400	15
Tomato paste	82	3.4	0.4	18.6	27	70	3.5	38	888	20			3300	49
Tomato puree	39	1.7	0.2	8.9	13	34	1.7	399	426	20			1600	3.3

6. DRY BEANS, PEAS and NUTS

low stress

| Food | Food Energy Calories | Basic Food Elements | | | | MINERALS (Milligrams) | | | | | | | | | VITAMINS | |
		Protein	Fat	Carbo-hydrates	Cal-cium	Phos-phorus	Iron	So-dium	Potas-sium	Magne-sium	Manga-nese	Zinc	Vitamin A	Vitamin C
Beans														
Lima, cooked	138	8.2	0.6	25.6	29	154	3.1	2	612			0.9		
Mung, sprouted, cooked	28	3.2	tr.	5.6	16.8	48	0.88	4	156				24	6.4
Pinto, dry	349	22.9	1.2	63.7	135	457	6.4	10	984					
Snap green, cooked	24	1.6	tr.	5.6	50.4	37	0.6	4	151	32		0.3	544	12
Lentils														
cooked	106	7.8	0	19.3	25	119	2.1	—	249				20	
raw	340	24.7	1.1	60.1	79	377	6.8	30	790	80			60	

HIGH STRESS

Food	Basic Food Elements						MINERALS (Milligrams)						VITAMINS	
	Food Energy Calories	Protein	Fat	Carbo-hydrates	Cal-cium	Phos-phorus	Iron	So-dium	Potas-sium	Magne-sium	Manga-nese	Zinc	Vitamin A	Vitamin C
Nuts														
Almonds	598	18.6	54.2	19.5	234	504	4.7	4	**773**	270				
Peanuts, boiled	564	26.0	47.5	18.6	69	401	2.1	5	**674**	206				
Pinole	635	13.0	60.5	20.5	12	**604**	5.2						30	10
Nuts														
Brazil	646	14.4	65.9	11.0	186	**693**	**6.8**	1	670	225				
Butternuts	629	23.7	61.2	8.4	—	—		—	—	—				
Cashew	561	17.2	45.7	29.3	38	373	3.8	15	**464**	267			100	
Chestnuts	191	2.8	1.5	41.5	29	87	1.7	2	**410**					
Filberts (hazelnuts)	647	10.7	63.3	20	253	320	3.3	0.7	**473**				106.7	7.3
Hickory nuts	673	14	67.3	13.3	—	—	**2.7**	—	—					
Macadamia	692	7.8	71.7	15.9	48.1	161.1	2.0	—	**264**	—				
Peanuts														
raw	565	25.9	47.4	18.6	69.1	400.2	2.1	5.1	**674.7**	175				
roasted, salted	586	26.0	49.7	18.8	74.2	401.5	2.1	418.4	**674.7**	175				
roasted, unsalted	581	26.2	48.8	20.6	71.9	407.4	2.2	5.1	**699.6**	175		3.0		
Pecans	688	9.2	71.3	14.6	73.1	289.3	2.4		**603.6**	142			130.2	1.5
Pistachio	594	19.3	53.8	19.0	131.1	500.5	7.3		**973**	—			229.6	
Walnuts, black	628	20.7	59.6	15.1	—	**570**	6.0	3	460	190			302	
Walnuts, english	654	15.0	64.4	15.6	83	380	2.1	2	**450**	131			30	3
Soybeans	403	34.1	17.7	33.5	226	554	8.4	5	**1677**	265			80	

7. FRUIT and FRUIT PRODUCTS

Food	Food Energy Calories	Basic Food Elements Protein	Fat	Carbo-hydrates	Cal-cium	Phos-phorus	MINERALS (Milligrams) Iron	So-dium	Potas-sium	Magne-sium	Manga-nese	Zinc	VITAMINS Vitamin A	Vitamin C
low stress														
Acerola cherry, raw	28	.4	.3	6.8	12	11	.2	8	83					**1300**
Apple, raw unpared	58	0.2	0.6	14.5	7	10	0.3	1	110	8	.04	.1	90	4
Apricots														
dried, uncooked	260	5.0	0.5	66.5	67	108	5.5	26	**979**				**10,900**	12
raw	51	1.0	0.2	12.8	17	23	.5	1	**281**	12			**2700**	10
Avocado	167	2.1	16.4	6.3	10	42	0.6	3	**604**	45	0.59		290	14
Blackberries	58	1.2	0.9	12.9	32	19	0.9	1	**170**	30	3.4		200	21
Blueberries	62	0.7	0.5	15.3	15	13	1.0	1	**81**	10			100	14
Cantaloupe	30	0.7	0.1	7.5	14	16	0.4	12	**251**	16			**3400**	33
Cherries, sweet	70	1.3	0.3	17.4	22	19	0.4	2	**191**				110	
Coconut, fresh meat	346	3.5	35.3	9.4	13	95	1.7	23	**256**	46				3
Currants, red or white	50	1.4	0.2	12.1	32	23	1.0	2	**257**				120	41
Dates, dry, pitted	274	2.2	0.5	72.9	59	63	3.0	1	**648**	58			50	
Elderberries	72	2.6	(0.5)	16.4	38	28	1.6	—	**300**	—			**600**	36
Figs														
dried	274	4.3	1.3	69.1	126	77	3.0	34	**640**	71			80	
raw	80	1.2	0.3	20.3	35	22	0.6	2	**194**	20			80	2
Grapes														
American	69	1.3	1.0	15.7	16	12	0.4	3	**158**	13			100	4
European	67	0.6	0.3	17.3	12	20	0.4	3	**173**	6			100	4
Honeydew	33	0.8	0.3	7.7	14	16	0.4	12	**251**	18			40	23
Mangos	66	.7	.4	16.8	10	13	.4	7	**189**				**4800**	35

Food	Basic Food Elements				MINERALS (Milligrams)								VITAMINS	
	Food Energy Calories	Protein	Fat	Carbo-hydrates	Cal-cium	Phos-phorus	Iron	So-dium	Potas-sium	Magne-sium	Manga-nese	Ainc	Vitamin A	Vitamin C
Nectarines	64	.6		17.1	4	24	.5	6	294	13			1650	13
Papayas	39	.6	.1	10.	20	16	.3	3	234				1750	56
Peaches														
dried	262	3.1	0.7	68.3	48	117	6.0	16	950	10	0.11	0.2	3900	18
raw	38	0.6	0.1	9.7	9	19	0.5	1	202				1330	7
Pears														
dried	126	1.5	0.8	31.7	16	23	0.6	3	269	5	0.06	0.16	30	2
raw	61	0.7	0.4	15.3	8	11	0.3	2	130				20	4
Prunes	75	0.8	0.2	19.7	12	18	0.5	1	170	40			300	4
Pumpkin	26	1.0	0.1	6.5	21	44	0.8	1	340	12			1600	9
Raisins	289	2.5	0.2	77.4	62	101	3.5	27	763	35			20	1
Raspberries														
black	73	1.5	1.4	15.7	30	22	0.9	1	199					18
red	57	1.2	0.5	13.6	22	22	0.9	1	168				130	25
Strawberries	37	0.7	0.5	8.4	21	21	1.0	1	164	12	0.06		60	59
Watermelon	26	0.5	0.2	6.4	7	10	0.5	1	100	8			590	7
HIGH STRESS														
Bananas	85	1.1	0.2	22.2	8	26	0.7	1	370	33		0.2	190	10
Cherries, sour	58	1.2	0.3	14.3	22	19	0.4	2	191				1000	10
Grapefruit	41	0.5	0.09	10.6	16.2	16.2	0.4	0.9	135				81.1	37.8
Limes	28	0.7	0.2	9.5	33	18	0.6	2	102				10	37
Oranges	49	1.0	0.2	12.2	41	20	0.4	1	200	11	0.03	0.17	200	50
Pineapple	52	0.4	0.2	13.7	17	8	0.5	1	146	13			70	17

8. CEREAL GRAINS and GRAIN PRODUCTS

Food	Food Energy Calories	Basic Food Elements					Minerals (Milligrams)						Vitamins	
		Protein	Fat	Carbo-hydrates	Cal-cium	Phos-phorus	Iron	So-dium	Potas-sium	Magne-sium	Manga-nese	Zinc	Vitamin A	Vitamin C
low stress														
Barley, pearled	350	8	1	79	16	**189**	2.0	3	160	37				
Bread, whole wheat	240	12	4	48	100	228	3.2	**527**	273	78		1.8		
Buckwheat, dark flour	333	11.7	2.5	72.0	33	347	2.8	1	**656**					
Buckwheat, light flour	347	6.4	1.2	79.5	11	88	1.0	1	**320**					
Carob flour	180	4.5	1.4	80.7	**352**	81								
Millet	325	9.8	2.9	72.4	20		6.7		**427**					
Oatmeal	390	14.25	7.4	68.2	52.5	**405**	4.5	2	327.5	144		3.4		
Rye Wafers	346	15.4	tr.	77	53.9	388	3.8	**882**	600					
Wheat bran	213	16.0	4.6	61.9	119	**1276**	14.9	9	1121	490		9.8		
Wheat germ	360	27	11	47	70	1118	9.0	3	827	336		14.3		
Wheat shredded	360	8	4	80	44	**388**	3.6	3	348	133		2.8		
HIGH STRESS														
Crackers														
graham	385	8.0	9.4	73.4	40	149	1.5	**671**	385	51		1.1		
saltines	434	9.0	12	71.6	21	90	1.2	**1102**	120			0.5		
soda	440	9.2	13.1	70.7	22	89	1.5	**1100**	120	29				
whole wheat	404	8.4	13.8	68.3	23	190	0.3	**548**	190					
Macaroni	370	12.5	1.2	75.0	26.8	161.7	1.3	2.0	**196.7**	48		1.5		
Yeast, baker's compressed	86	12.1	0.4	11.0	13.0	394	4.9	16.1	**610.8**	59				

9. FATS and OILS

Food	Food Energy Calories	Basic Food Elements Protein	Fat	Carbo-hydrates	Cal-cium	Phos-phorus	MINERALS (Milligrams) Iron	So-dium	Potas-sium	Magne-sium	Manga-nese	Zinc	VITAMINS Vitamin A	Vitamin C

HIGH STRESS

Food	Food Energy Calories	Protein	Fat	Carbo-hydrates	Cal-cium	Phos-phorus	Iron	So-dium	Potas-sium	Magne-sium	Manga-nese	Zinc	Vitamin A	Vitamin C
Cornstarch	362	0.31	trace	87.7	0	0	0	trace	trace	0		0	0	0
Cottonseed oil	885	0	100	0	0	0	0	0	0	0		0	0	0
Gravy, meat, brown	205	1.5	17.5	10.0	trace	0	0.5	*	10					
Mayonnaise	721	1.1	80.0	2.1	21.4	28.6	0.07	599	35.7				278	
Mustard, yellow, prepared	75	4.7	4.4	6.4	83.8	72.8	2.0	1250	129.8	48				
Shortening, vegetable	879	—	98.6	—	0	0	0	—	—	—			0	0

* = Sodium content is largely dependent upon salt added in preparation and cooking

10. SUGARS, SWEETS and SYRUPS

HIGH STRESS

Food	Food Energy Calories	Protein	Fat	Carbo-hydrates	Cal-cium	Phos-phorus	Iron	So-dium	Potas-sium	Magne-sium	Manga-nese	Zinc	Vitamin A	Vitamin C
Cane syrup	284	0.5	0.2	72.6	70	42	1.2		445					3
Honey, strained	306	0.2	0	78.0	20	16	0.8	5	51	3				1
Maple syrup	250	0	0	64.0	165	15	1.0	15	130					
Molasses, Blackstrap	27			6.8	85	10	2	12	365	32				
Sorghum syrup	260			13.4	30	5	2.4	4	120					

11. FOOD JUICES, BEVERAGES

Food	Food Energy Calories	Basic Food Elements			Minerals (Milligrams)								Vitamins	
		Protein	Fat	Carbo-hydrates	Cal-cium	Phos-phorus	Iron	So-dium	Potas-sium	Magne-sium	Manga-nese	Zinc	Vitamin A	Vitamin C
low stress														
Food Juices														
Acerola	23	.4	.3	4.8	**10**	9	.5	3	**101**	4		.05		**1600**
Apple	47	.1		11.9	6	9	.6	1	**341**	23				1
Carrot	42	1.1	.2	9.7	37	36	.7	47	**341**	22		0.4	**11,000**	8
Celery	17	.9	.1	3.9	39	28	.3	126			0.16		240	9
Grape	66	.2	trace	16.6	11	12	.3	2	**116**	12				
Pear/Carrot														
Pear	52	0.4	0.2	7.6	4	5.5	0.2	1	65	2.5	0.03	0.08	10	2
Carrot	52	0.6	0.1	4.8	18.5	18	0.4	23.5	170	11.5		0.2	5500	4
TOTALS		1.0	0.3	12.4	22.5	23.5	0.6	24.5	**235**	14.0	0.03	0.28	**5510**	6
Pear/Celery														
Pear	39	0.4	0.2	7.6	4	5.5	0.2	1	65	2.5	0.03	0.08	10	2
Celery	39	0.5	0.05	1.9	19.5	14	0.15	63	170	11	0.08		120	4.5
TOTALS		0.9	0.25	9.5	23.5	19.5	0.35	64	**235**	13.5	0.11	0.08	130	6.5
HIGH STRESS														
Coffee, instant	98.1	trace	trace	trace	2	4	.1	1	**36**					
Food Juices														
Orange	**45**		**.2**	**10.2**	**11**	**17**	**.2**	1	**200**	11		.02	200	50
Pineapple, unsweetened	55	.4	.1	13.5	15	9	.3	1	**149**	12			50	9
Tomato juice canned	19	.9	.1	4.3	7	18	.9	200	**227**	10			**800**	16

Understanding BLOOD PRESSURE DRUGS

Any drug effect other than what is therapeutically intended can be called a side effect. It may be expected and benign, or unexpected and potentially harmful. . . . A side effect may be tolerated for a necessary therapeutic effect or it may be hazardous and unacceptable, and require discontinuation of the drug. . . . Most important, patients need to be told what side effects to expect so they won't become worried or even stop taking the drug on their own.

Nurse's Guide To Drugs/page 19
Intermed Communications, Inc.

Diuretics

This listing comprises the most popularly prescribed diuretics. There are other diuretic name brands on the market. All have similar side effects. Ask your physician for a Description Sheet on the drug or drugs he is prescribing for you. For much of the terminology used under the heading Side Effects . . . you will need a medical dictionary to understand the meaning of the medical words. A good medical dictionary is Taber's Cyclopedic Medical Dictionary. It can be found in most bookstores and is an economical and sound investment.

NAME	Possible SIDE EFFECTS	Other CONSIDERATIONS
[1] **Diuretics**		
acetazolamide Diamox Hydrazol	Bone marrow depression, abnormal decrease in number of blood platelets, abnormal decrease of white blood corpuscles, extremely low levels of white blood cell count. High fever, mouth, rectal and vagina ulcers. Abnormal sensations . . . numbness, prickling, tingling. Drowsiness, confusion, depression, dizziness, ringing in the ears. Diarrhea, weight loss, loss of appetite, nausea, constipation, dry mouth, excessive thirst. Excessive urination, disturbance in acid balance of the body, muscular weakness, rash, severe itching.	Should be used cautiously in emphysema, chronic lung disease or if patient is using other diuretics. High-potassium diet should be considered.

---

[1] Diuretics increase the urinary excretion of water and sodium. Some diuretics begin to act within 1 to 3 hours after taking. This action may last 8 to 12 hours. Timed-release drugs can last as long as 24 hours. If the diuretic is administered intravenously, diuretic action can begin within 2 minutes and will last up to 5 hours. Often, the first drug prescribed for high blood pressure . . . is a diuretic that promotes loss of water, sodium and potassium. Since potassium loss is undesirable, diuretics are frequently combined with potassium supplements.

NAME	Possible SIDE EFFECTS	Other CONSIDERATIONS
bendroflu-methiazide Naturetin	Abnormal decrease of white blood cor-puscles. Extremely low levels of white blood cell count with high fever, and pos-sible mouth, rectal and vagina ulcers. Dizziness, abnormal sensations . . . numbness, prickling, tingling. Headache, weakness, temporary blurred vision. Loss of appetite, irritable stomach, diar-rhea, constipation. Extreme potassium de-pletion, increase in blood sugar (as in diabetes), hemorrhages into the skin, fever, muscle spasm.	Should not be used in kidney failure. Watch for signs of potassium loss. Give in morning.
benzthiazide Aquapres Aquasec, Aquastat, Aquatag, Di-retic, Diucen, Hydrex, Lema-zide, Marazide, Proaqua, Rid-ema, S-Aqua, Urazide	Abnormal decrease of white blood cor-puscles. Extremely low levels of white blood cell count with high fever and pos-sible mouth, rectal and vagina ulcers, de-pletion of red blood cells in bone marrow. Dizziness, difficulty in maintaining bal-ance, headache, weakness, blurred vision, objects appear to be yellow, loss of appetite, stomach distress, nausea, cramps, diarrhea, constipation, potassium imbalance, rash, fever, incrèased irrita-bility with possible convulsions.	Should not be used in kid-ney failure. Watch for signs of potassium loss. Give in morning.
chlorothiazide Diuril Ro-Chlorozide	Abnormal decrease of white blood cor-puscles. Extremely low levels of white blood cell count with high fever, and pos-sible mouth, rectal and vagina ulcers. De-pletion of red blood cells in bone marrow. Headache, loss of balance, dizziness, weakness. Blurred vision, objects appear to be yellow. Loss of appetite, stomach distress, nausea, vomiting, cramps, diar-rhea, constipation. Abnormal amount of sugar in urine. Critical loss of potassium, gout, skin rash, fever, muscle spasms and increased irritability with possible convulsions.	Should not be used in kid-ney failure. Watch for signs of potassium loss. Avoid I.V. infiltration: can be very painful. Give in morning.
furosemide Lasix	Diminished blood supply with excessive passage of urine, anemia, abnormal de-crease of white blood corpuscles. Ex-tremely low levels of white blood cell count with high fever and possible mouth, rectal, vagina ulcers. Weakness, fatigue, lethargy. Light-headedness, tin-gling. Ringing in the ears, hearing impair-ment (in I.V. administration), blurred vision. Thirst, nausea, vomiting, diar-rhea, stomach pains. Urinary bladder spasm, dehydration, potassium depletion, itching skin, muscle cramps and sweating.	Should not be used in kid-ney failure nor in potas-sium imbalance. Give in morning.

NAME	Possible SIDE EFFECTS	Other CONSIDERATIONS
hydrochloro-thiazide Chloride, Delco-Retic, Diu-Scrip, Esidrix, Hydro-Diuril, Hydromal, Hydro-Z-25 (50), Hype-etic, Kenazide, Lexor, Oretic, Ro-Hydrazide, Zide	Abnormal decrease of white blood corpuscles. Extremely low levels of white blood cell count with high fever and possible mouth, rectal and vagina ulcers. Loss of balance, dizziness. Abnormal sensations . . . numbness, prickling, tingling. Headache, restlessness, weakness. Blurred vision, objects appear to be yellow. Loss of appetite, irritable stomach, nausea, diarrhea, cramps, constipation. Skin rash, hemorrhages into the skin. Jaundice, fever, muscle spasm.	Should not be used in kidney failure nor in potassium imbalance. Give in morning.
spironolactone Aldactone	Confusion, headache, drowsiness, muscular incoordination, dry mouth, thirst, diarrhea. Dehydration. Skin rashes, drug fever, abnormally large mammary glands in the male; sometimes may secrete milk. Decreased sex drive in male, impotence, irregular menses, absence or suppression of menstruation. Post-menopausal bleeding. Excessive growth of hair or hair growth in unusual places, deepened voice.	Should not be used in kidney failure. Use cautiously in potassium imbalance. This is a potassium-sparing diuretic. Diuretic effect delayed 2-3 days when used alone. Patient should avoid excessive intake of potassium-rich foods. Breast cancer reported in some people taking spironolactone.
trichlor-methiazide Aquazide, Aquex, Diurese, Methahydrin, Naqua, Rochlomethiazide	Abnormal decrease of white blood corpuscles. Extremely low levels of white blood cell count with high fever and possible mouth, rectal and vagina ulcers. Loss of balance, dizziness. Abnormal sensations . . . numbness, prickling, tingling. Headache, weakness, restlessness. Temporary blurred vision, objects appear to be yellow. Loss of appetite, stomach irritation, cramps, nausea, vomiting, diarrhea, constipation. Potassium imbalance. Hemorrhages into the skin, skin rash, jaundice, fever, increased irritability with possible convulsions, muscle spasm.	Should not be used in kidney failure or severe kidney disease. Watch for signs of potassium loss. Monitor blood sugar. Give in morning.

Potassium Replacement Drugs

Potassium is an electrolyte which is essential to many body processes. Long-term use of diuretics may cause an excessive loss of potassium! Heart patients are quite sensitive to potassium deficiency. Often a Potassium Replacement supplement is given by a doctor when diuretics cause severe Potassium losses. Because excessive Potassium levels can also be hazardous, the doctor must monitor this carefully.

NAME	Possible SIDE EFFECTS	Other CONSIDERATIONS
Potassium Replacement		
potassium bi-carbonate K-Lyte, K-Lyte DS	Abnormal sensations . . . numbness, prickling, tingling. Mental confusion, weakness, heaviness of legs. Possible fall in blood pressure, irregular heart rhythm, possible cardiac arrest. Nausea, stomach pains, diarrhea, hemorrhage, diminished amount of urine formation, cold skin.	Should not be used in severe kidney disorder. Use with caution in heart disease. Never switch potassium products without a doctor's orders.
potassium chloride K-Lor, K-Lyte/ C1, K-10, Kao-chlor, S-F 10%, Kaon, Kato Powder, Kay-Ciel, Klor-10%, Kloride, Klo-trix, Klorvess, Pfiklor, Slow K	Abnormal sensations . . . numbness, prickling, tingling. Mental confusion, heaviness of legs, listlessness. Irregular heart rhythm, possible cardiac arrest. Nausea, stomach pain, diarrhea, possible ulcers, diminished amount of urine formation, cold skin.	Should not be used in severe kidney disorder. Use with caution in heart disease. Never switch potassium products without doctor's orders. In I.V. . . . must be given slowly.

There are other potassium replacement drugs. Ask your physician for a Description Sheet on the drug or drugs he is prescribing for you. All have similar side effects.

Antihypertensive drugs are used to treat those with high blood pressure . . . from mild to severe conditions. There are approximately 10 different types of drugs. Some affect the central sympathetic nervous system . . . others relax the arterial muscles. Some drugs are blocking agents affecting renin. Renin is an enzyme made, stored and secreted by the kidneys. It is believed to play a significant role in maintaining blood pressure.

No single drug is ideal in preventing high blood pressure. All have potential side effects.

NAME	Possible SIDE EFFECTS	Other CONSIDERATIONS
Antihypertensives		
alseroxylon Raudolfin, Rautensin, Rauwiloid, Vio-Serpine	Depression, drowsiness, mental confusion, anxiety, nervousness, nightmares, fatigue. Nasal stuffiness, dry mouth, glaucoma. Nausea, vomiting, gastrointestinal bleeding, severe itching, rash, impotence, water retention and weight gain.	Use cautiously in patients with severe heart or other vascular disease, peptic ulcer, colitis, kidney disease, gallstones, mental disorders or those undergoing surgery. Female patients should notify doctor if she becomes pregnant. Give drug with meals. Do not discontinue this drug suddenly. Watch for mental depression.
captopril Capoten	Skin rash with severe itching. Facial swelling. Low blood pressure. Abnormal rapidity of heart action, heart palpitations, angina, mycardial infarction, congestive heart failure, spasms of blood vessels (Raynaud's syndrome). Loss of taste or taste impairment. Weight loss, stomach irritation, abdominal pain, nausea, vomiting, diarrhea, loss of appetite. Constipation, ulcers, dizziness, headache, fatigue, insomnia. Dry mouth, labored breathing. Abnormal sensations . . . numbness, prickling, tingling.	Should be taken one hour before meals. If possible, discontinue the patient's previous antihypertensive drugs for one week before starting captopril. Patients with impaired kidney function may respond to smaller or less frequent doses.
clonidine hydrochloride Catapres	Dizziness, fatigue, drowsiness, behavioral changes, nightmares, headache, nervousness. Dry mouth, constipation, urinary retention, impotence.	Use cautiously in patients with severe heart or other vascular disease, chronic kidney problems, history of depression, or those taking other antihypertensives. Do not discontinue abruptly. Last dose should be taken immediately before retiring.

NAME	Possible SIDE EFFECTS	Other CONSIDERATIONS
cryptenamine acetate Unitensen Aqueous	Mental confusion, irregular heart rhythm. Blurred vision, unpleasant taste, excessive salivation. Nausea, vomiting, burning in esophagus, hiccups, bronchial constriction.	Use cautiously in patients with angina, cerebrovascular disease, bronchial asthma, kidney insufficiency. The range between therapeutic and toxic doses of this drug is narrow.
diazoxide Hyperstat (I.V. only) Proglem, Proglycem	Abnormal decrease of white blood corpuscles, flushing, dizziness, light-headedness, euphoria. Sodium and water retention, angina, low blood pressure, irregular heart rhythm. Nausea, vomiting, stomach pain. Decreased urinary output. Rash, labored breathing, choking sensation, fever.	Use cautiously in patients with severe heart or other vascular disease. This drug may alter a diabetic's insulin requirements.
guanethidine sulfate Ismelin	Weakness, dizziness, irregular heart rhythm, congestive heart failure. Nasal stuffiness, dry mouth, water retention, weight gain, diarrhea. In the male, an inability to ejaculate.	Use cautiously in patients with severe heart or other vascular disease, peptic ulcer, impaired kidney function, bronchial asthma, or those taking other antihypertensives. Do not discontinue this drug suddenly.
hydralazine hydrochloride Apresoline Dralzine, Hydralyn, Nor-Pres 25, Rolazine	Abnormal decrease of white blood corpuscles and in number of blood platelets. Headache, neuritis, dizziness. Irregular heart rhythm, angina, palpitations, sodium retention, Nausea, vomiting, loss of appetite, diarrhea. Skin rash, lupus erythematosus, weight gain.	Use cautiously in patients with severe heart disease or those taking other antihypertensive drugs. Do not discontinue this drug suddenly. Give drug with meals to increase absorption.
mecamylamine hydrochloride Inversine	Blurred vision. Abnormal sensations . . . numbness, prickling, tingling. Tremors, fatigue, convulsions, dizziness, weakness, psychic changes. Dry mouth, inflammation of the tongue. Loss of appetite, nausea, vomiting, constipation, diarrhea. Urinary retention, impotence or decreased sex drive.	Not to be used in patients with heart disease, uremia. Use cautiously in patients with kidney insufficiency, glaucoma, vscular disease or those taking other antihypertensive drugs.
methyldopa Aldomet	Abnormal decrease in number of blood platelets. Headache, dizziness, decreased mental acuity, psychic disturbances, depression, weakness, loss of strength. Angina, heart inflammation. Nasal stuffiness, dry mouth, diarrhea. Impotence, skin rash, fever, anemia.	Use cautiously in patients taking other antihypertensive drugs. Urine may turn dark in toilet bowls treated with bleach. Do not stop drug suddenly.

NAME	Possible SIDE EFFECTS	Other CONSIDERATIONS
metoprolol tartrate Lopressor	Abnormal decrease in number of blood platelets. Depression, giddiness, hallucinations, drowsiness, visual disturbances. Congestive heart failure, angina, heart attack, low blood pressure, shock. Skin rash, wheezing, asthma.	Use cautiously in patients with heart disease, diabetes, respiratory diseases or those taking other antihypertensive drugs. Check pulse rate before giving drug. If less than 60 beats a minute . . . hold drug and call doctor immediately.
pargyline hydrochloride Eutonyl	Convulsions, tremors, psychic changes, nightmares, hyperexcitability, dizziness, fainting, drowsiness. Dry mouth, eye damage. Nausea, vomiting, increase appetite. Fluid retention, hypoglycemia, impotence.	Not to be used in those with advanced kidney failure or Parkinson's disease or those who are hyperactive or hyperexcitable. Use cautiously in patients receiving other antihypertensives or who have liver disease. Periodic eye examinations advisable. Patient should be warned not to take any other medications, including over-the-counter cold remedies . . . without doctor's approval. Avoid eating aged cheese, sour cream, figs, raisins, chicken livers, chocolate, caffeine products or cola drinks.
prazosin hydrochloride Minipress	Headache, dizziness, drowsiness, weakness, depression. Heart palpitations. Blurred vision. Vomiting, diarrhea, stomach cramps, dry mouth, constipation.	Use cautiously in patients using other antihypertensive drugs. If initial dose is greater than 1 mg., patient may have a temporary loss of consciousness due to inadequate flow of blood to the brain. Drug should not be discontinued abruptly.
propranolol hydrochloride Inderal	Abnormal decrease in number of blood platelets. Extremely low levels of white blood cell count. High fever with possible mouth, rectal and vagina ulcers. Depression, giddiness, hallucinations, visual disturbances. Congestive heart failure, loss of consciousness, shock. Nausea, vomiting, diarrhea. Skin rash, wheezing, asthma.	Do not use in diabetes, asthma, heart problems or during ethyl ether anesthesia. Do not discontinue abruptly. Take with meals.

NAME	Possible SIDE EFFECTS	Other CONSIDERATIONS
rauwolfia serpentina HBP, Hiwolfia, Hyper-Rauw, Hywolfia, Rau, Raudixin, Rauja, Raumason, Rauneed, Raupoid, Rauserpa, Rauserpin, Rausertina, Rauval, Rauwoldin, Rawfola, Ru-Hy-T, Serifa, Serfolia, T-Rau Wolfina	Depression, mental confusion, anxiety, nervousness, nightmares, headache. Dry mouth, nasal stuffiness, glaucoma. Nausea, vomiting, gastrointestinal bleeding. Skin rash, severe itching. Water retention, weight gain, impotence.	Do not use in patients with depression. Use cautiously in patients with heart disease, impaired kidney function, peptic ulcer, colitis, gallstones, or those taking other antihypertensive drugs. Do not discontinue abruptly. Female patient should notify doctor if she becomes pregnant. Notify doctor immediately if you have nightmares.
rescinnamine Anaprel Cinnasil Moderil	Depression, mental confusion, drowsiness, nervousness, anxiety, nightmares. Dry mouth, nasal stuffiness, glaucoma. Nausea, vomiting, gastrointestinal bleeding. Skin rash, severe itching. Water retention, weight gain, impotence.	Do not use in patients with depression. Use cautiously in patients with heart disease, impaired kidney function, peptic ulcer, colitis, gallstones, or those taking other antihypertensive drugs. Do not discontinue abruptly. Female patient should notify doctor if she becomes pregnant. Notify doctor immediately if you have nightmares.
reserpine Alkarau, Arcum R-S, Bonapene, Broserpine, De Serpa, Elserpine, Geneserp #2, Hiserpia, Hyperine, Maso-Serpine, Rauloydin, Raurine, Rau-Sed, Rauserpin, Relerserp-5, Reserjen, Reserpaneed, Reserpoid, Rolserp, Sandril, Serp, Serpalan, Serpena, Serpanray, Serpasil, Serpasil, Serpate, Sertabs, Sertina, Tensin, T-Serp, Tri-Serp, Vio-Serpine, Zepine	Depression, mental confusion, drowsiness, nervousness, anxiety, nightmares. Dry mouth, nasal stuffiness, glaucoma. Hyperacidity, nausea, vomiting, gastrointestinal bleeding, gall bladder colic. Skin rash, severe itching. Water retention, weight gain, impotence.	Do not use in patients with depression. Use cautiously in patients with heart disease, impaired kidney function, peptic ulcer, colitis, gallstones, or those taking other antihypertensive drugs. Do not discontinue abruptly. Female patient should notify doctor if she becomes pregnant. Notify doctor immediately if you have nightmares.

The Medical Approach versus The Nutritional Approach

ARLIGHTHRITIS (including LUPUS) ①
by Salem Kirban

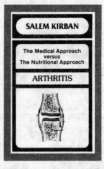

What causes arthritis? How many types of arthritis are there? Does medicine help or hinder? Is chiropractic treatment valid? How will the disease progress if not corrected? What do physicians recommend? What is the nutritional approach to the same problem? How is **Lupus** treated medically, nutritionally?

How to recognize the symptoms of arthritis. What diet do many nutritionists feel is beneficial? What foods should I avoid? Answers to these and more!

The Medical Approach versus The Nutritional Approach

CANCER
(including Breast and Lung) ②
by Salem Kirban

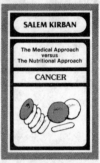

What causes cancer? What do nutritionists believe is the cause of cancer? What are the basic types of cancer? Is surgery the answer? What about chemotherapy? Can drugs cure cancer? What side effects can I expect?

Is a proper nutrition program effective against cancer? What foods should I eat? Should I go on a juice diet?

The Medical Approach versus The Nutritional Approach

HEART DISEASE ③
by Salem Kirban

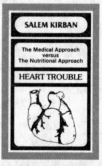

Does a diagnosis of heart trouble mean the end is near? Can I do something about it and live a happy, healthy long life . . . even after a heart attack?

What about drugs and Vitamin E? What is the sensible nutritional approach to the problem? How can I regain a sense of well-being and abundant energy without fear? What foods should I avoid? How can I flush my system clean again?

The Medical Approach versus The Nutritional Approach

HIGH BLOOD PRESSURE ④
by Salem Kirban

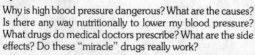

Why is high blood pressure dangerous? What are the causes? Is there any way nutritionally to lower my blood pressure? What drugs do medical doctors prescribe? What are the side effects? Do these "miracle" drugs really work?

What is the nutritional approach to high blood pressure? What juices should I drink? What vitamins and minerals are beneficial? Is fasting beneficial? What foods should I eat?

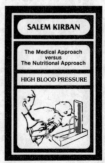

The Medical Approach versus The Nutritional Approach

DIABETES
by Salem Kirban ⑤

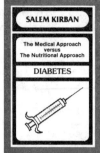

What causes diabetes? Must I change my lifestyle? Why do medical doctors prescribe insulin? What is the prognosis for one who is told he has diabetes?

Can a supervised nutrition program minimize the effect of diabetes? Will it provide a normal lifestyle? What foods should you eat? What juices are beneficial? Does the water I drink make a difference? Are vitamins and minerals and herbs worthwhile?

The Medical Approach versus The Nutritional Approach

BOWEL PROBLEMS
by Salem Kirban ⑥

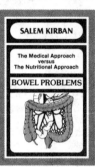

How can I unlock my bowels for better health? How can I achieve that vibrant vitality again and gain that schoolgirl complexion? How can I break the laxative habit? Are drugs the answer?

How can I get rid of hemorrhoids forever? What vitamins and juices are especially beneficial? Are suppositories worthwhile? If so, what type? Can you have daily bowel movements and still be constipated?

The Medical Approach versus The Nutritional Approach

PROSTATE PROBLEMS
by Salem Kirban ⑦

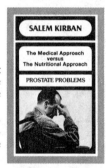

What are the early warning signs of prostate problems? What drugs do medical doctors recommend? What are the side effects? What surgery do they recommend? Is the cure worse than the problem?

Does the nutritional approach offer a more lasting alternative? What diet is recommended? How can you avoid prostate problems in sexual union? Why waiting to correct the problem is dangerous! Do juices and vitamins help?

The Medical Approach versus The Nutritional Approach

ULCERS
by Salem Kirban ⑧

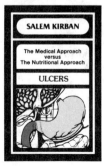

What causes gastric and duodenal ulcers? Are the "miracle" drugs really effective or do they bring with them a host of insidious side effects? What warning signals give you advance notice of an impending ulcer?

What foods are especially helpful? Are juices beneficial? Which ones and how should they be taken? What may happen if you don't change your way of life? What vitamins, minerals are beneficial?

The Medical Approach versus The Nutritional Approach
KIDNEY DISEASE
by Salem Kirban

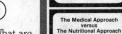

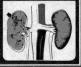

What is the medical approach to kidney disease? What are some of the problems that can develop if the disease is not nipped in the bud? What are the side effects of the drugs prescribed?

Is meat harmful? What type of diet is beneficial? Is a supervised fast recommended? How long? What common, ordinary foods and juices have proven beneficial? What vitamins and minerals help? What about herbs?

The Medical Approach versus The Nutritional Approach
EYESIGHT
by Salem Kirban
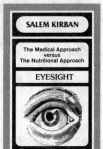

Are glasses the answer to failing eyesight? Is the medical approach to Cataracts the only solution? What do nutritionists recommend?

What eye exercises may prove beneficial for my eyes? Can I throw away my glasses? Is poor eyesight an indication of other growing physical problems? Can diet correct my poor eyesight? What juices may prove beneficial? What combination of vitamins and minerals should I take?

The Medical Approach versus The Nutritional Approach
IMPOTENCE/ FRIGIDITY
by Salem Kirban
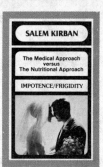

Impotence is the incapacity of the male to have sexual union. Frigidity is the incapacity of the female for sexual response. Both of these problems are growing because of today's stressful lifestyle! They lead to other trials!

What is the medical approach to these problems? How successful are they? What is the nutritional approach? What type of diet is recommended? Do juices help? Are herbs beneficial? Much more!

The Medical Approach versus The Nutritional Approach
COLITIS/CROHN'S DISEASE
by Salem Kirban
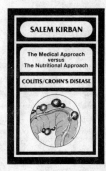

What causes Colitis? What drugs do doctors recommend? What are the side effects: How successful is surgery? What is the nutritional approach to Colitis? What foods are beneficial? What about juices and vitamins?

What is Crohn's Disease? What are the symptoms? Why does it recur? What is the medical approach to the problem? What is the nutritional approach? Can juices and vitamins correct the cause?

HOW TO BE YOUR AGAIN (13)
by Salem Kirban

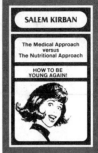

How can I restore my energy and eliminate fatigue? How can I develop Reserve Energy as an insurance to good health and a hedge against illness? How can I begin a simple, day by day health program?

How much should I eat and when should I eat? How can I check my own Nutrition Profile daily? How can I feel like 20 at age 60? How can I turn my marriage into a honeymoon again? When should I take vitamins, minerals? What juices are vital for a youthful life?

OBESITY (14)
by Salem Kirban

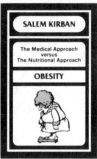

What causes Obesity? Why don't fad diets work? Is being overweight a glandular problem or a dietary problem? Is obesity a liver, pancreas or thyroid problem?

What is the medical approach to treating those who are overweight? What illnesses will obesity encourage? Why does the nutritionist treat your colon? What nutritional approach will take off weight easily and permanently giving you a new lease on life?

HEADACHES (15)
by Salem Kirban

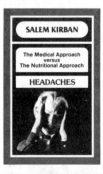

What causes headaches? Can headaches cause depression and hypoglycemia? Are women more prone to have nagging headaches? Must you live with migraine headaches all your life? What is the medical approach to headache problems?

Can a proper nutritional approach rid you of migraine headaches? Do vitamins help? Is fasting beneficial.? What about the pressure point techniques? What 3 herbs promise headache relief? How to tell your migraine *"Goodbye!"*

HYPOGLYCEMIA (16)
by Salem Kirban

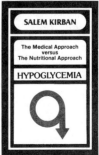

Is Hypoglycemia a fact or a fad? Why has this word . . . Hypoglycemia . . . become the focus of intense controversy? Is it the cause of many unexplained ills? What is the medical approach to this problem?

Anxiety, irritability, exhaustion, lack of sex drive, constant worrying, headaches, indecisiveness, insomnia, crying spells and forgetfulness . . . are these all signs of Hypoglycemia? How do nutritionists approach this problem with diet and supplements? Will this approach give you a new life?

ORDER FORM   **SALEM KIRBAN Health Books**

Quantity	Description	Price	Total
	The MEDICAL APPROACH Versus The NUTRITIONAL APPROACH Series		
_____	1 Arthritis	$ 5.00	_____
_____	2 Cancer	5.00	_____
_____	3 Heart Disease	5.00	_____
_____	4 High Blood Pressure	5.00	_____
_____	5 Diabetes	5.00	_____
_____	6 Bowel Problems	5.00	_____
_____	7 Prostate Problems	5.00	_____
_____	8 Ulcers	5.00	_____
_____	9 Kidney Disease	5.00	_____
_____	10 Eyesight	5.00	_____
_____	11 Impotence and Frigidity	5.00	_____
_____	12 Colitis/Crohn's Disease	5.00	_____
_____	13 How To Be Young Again	5.00	_____
_____	14 Obesity	5.00	_____
_____	15 Headaches	5.00	_____
_____	16 Hypoglycemia	5.00	_____
_____	**All 16 Health Books** _(Save $30)_	**$50.00**	_____

Single Book	$5	All 16 Books	$50*
Any 3 Books	$12	(*You save $30)	

Other SALEM KIRBAN HEALTH BOOKS

_____	Unlocking Your Bowels For Better Health	4.95	_____
_____	How Juices Restore Health Naturally	4.95	_____
_____	How To Eat Your Way Back To Vibrant Health	4.95	_____
_____	How To Keep Healthy & Happy By Fasting	4.95	_____
_____	The Getting Back To Nature Diet	4.95	_____
_____	**How To Win Over IMPOTENCE/FRIGIDITY**	6.95	_____
	(Expanded Version with Full Color Section)		

Total for Books _____
Shipping & Handling _____
Total Enclosed $ _____

(We do NOT invoice. Check must accompany order, please.)

☐ Check enclosed
☐ Master Charge
☐ VISA

When using Credit Card, show number in space below.

When Using MasterCard Also Give Interbank No. (Just above your name on card)

Card Ex- pires	Month	Year

*POSTAGE & HANDLING Use the easy chart to figure postage, shipping and handling charges. Send correct amount and avoid delay.

TOTAL FOR BOOKS	Up to 5.00	5.01- 10.00	10.01- 20.00	20.01- 35.00	Over 35.00
DELIVERY CHARGE	1.50	2.00	2.50	2.95	NO CHARGE

FOR ADDITIONAL SAVINGS: Orders Over $35.00 Are Now Postage-Free!

SHIP TO _____
　　　　Mr./Mrs./Miss　　　(Please PRINT)

Address _____

City _____ State _____ ZIP _____

SALEM KIRBAN, Inc./Kent Road, Huntingdon Valley, Pennsylvania 19006